Becoming a Student Midwife: The Book For Passionate Midwives In The Making

CW01335720

Ellie Durant

First Edition (E-book) May 2014

Second Revision (Paperback) October 2014

Becoming a Student Midwife:
The Book for Passionate Midwives in the Making

Copyright © Eleanor Durant, 2014

(ellie@midwifediaries.com)

About the Author:

Ellie Durant is a UK trained
midwife who has worked in
the NHS, and in New
Zealand.

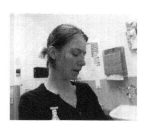

Ellie launched MidwifeDiaries.com in 2012 to offer
resources for midwives and midwives in the making.
The MidwifeDiaries Facebook page was formed and
is a fast growing, supportive environment for
applicants and students.

Ellie is passionate about creating high quality,
accessible resources written in plain English made
available to applicants, students, and qualified
midwives. She believes the most effective way to
achieve holistic midwifery care for women and
families is to ensure supportive, empowering
education for midwives.

Ellie currently lives and works as a midwifery writer in
Leicester, professionally collaborating with MTC
partnership and holistic careers adviser Jan Hyde.

'Becoming a Student Midwife' was published in May
2014 and quickly rose to be Amazon's best-selling
text on entry into midwifery.

Acknowledgements

Thanks so much to the wonderful community of midwives and midwives in the making who've supported MidwifeDiaries.com. This book would not have happened without you, and I'm so grateful.

Thankyou everyone else who helped. There are lots of you and you all know who you are! Thanks go especially to my Mum, Nicola, who was a neonatal nurse and who inspired me to be a midwife in the first place. Thanks to my Dad, Ian, for copy editing and making this book readable and coherent! Thank you careers adviser Jan Hyde for your encouragement, professional advice and insight.

Thanks most of all to my partner James, the unsung hero of Midwife Diaries. Without you I'd be lost, and with you I seem to be capable in ways which surprise me every day.

CONTENTS

Introduction 1

Your Journey Into Midwifery 1

First, Check Midwifery Is Right For You 4

How To Get The Most Out Of This Book 7

Chapter One: A Successful Application. 9

Choosing Your University 9

Successfully Applying Through UCAS 12

Entry Grades And How To Get Them 13

Getting Experience and Volunteering 15

Computer And Research Tricks 18

Chapter Two: Your Personal Statement 22

Introduction 22

The Basics 23

Personal Statement Example 1: Common Mistakes
.... 28

Personal Statement Example 1: Analysis 31

Personal Statement Example 2: Excellent
Technique 44

Personal Statement Example 2: Analysis 47

Personal Statement Example 3: Excellent
Technique From A 'Mature Student' 58

Personal Statement Example 3: Analysis 61

Chapter Three: Nervousness And How To Handle It 71

Introduction 71

Chronic Nervousness and Anxiety 73

Techniques and Using DOPE in Your Interview
.... 74

    Don't Fight With Your Emotions 74

    Neuro-Linguistic Programming 75

    Power Posing 77

    Equality Philosophy 79

Chapter Four: Panel Interview Technique 81

How To Dress And How To Show Your
Composure On Interview Day 81

Dress And Composure 82

Essential Knowledge 85

The 5 Questions You Should Prepare For 86

Research Your University 90

Use Of Humour 92

'Is There Anything You Want To Ask?' - How To
Question Your Interviewer 93

The Evening Before And Day Of Your Interview
.... 94

Chapter Five: Above And Beyond...... 96

What Else Interviewers Look For............................96

Your Specialist Interest Subject................................98

Some Resources For Learning About Your
Specialist Interest Subject Include… 100

Showing Your Resilience...104

Your Portfolio..106

Chapter Six: Additional Selection Activities 109

Group Interviews...110

Basics 110

Presentations 114

Numeracy Tests 117

Literacy Tests..119

Essay Exams..119

Chapter Seven: Practice Questions And Answers 124

Practice Numeracy Tests 124

Test One 124

Test Two..130

Practice Literacy Tests 135

Type 1: Essays...135

Type 2: Language Comprehension 135

Practice Panel Interview Questions 141

Questions On Your Personality And How You Will Cope With The Challenges Of The Course 143

Questions On Your Personal Opinions And Factual Knowledge About Midwifery And Related Topics..146

Scenario Based Questions 148

Answers To Numeracy Tests................................149

Test One 149

Test Two 154

Answers To Literacy Tests 159

Type 1: Essays...159

Type 2: Language Comprehension 162

Practice Panel Interview Answers 169

Analysis And Sample Answers: On Your Personality And How You Will Cope With The Challenges Of The Course 169

Analysis And Sample Answers: On Your Personal Opinions And Factual Knowledge About Midwifery And Related Topics 197

Analysis And Sample Answers: Scenario Based Questions..216

Chapter Eight: Male Midwives In The Making... 222

The Challenges You Might Face 222

Chapter Nine: If You Didn't Get Offered A Place This Year 229

If You Didn't Get Offered a Place This Year: What it Says About You and Your Chances of Success 229

Congratulations! 234

Introduction

Your Journey Into Midwifery

Hi, I'm Ellie, I'm a UK trained and qualified midwife who created MidwifeDiaries.com, the site that works to empower midwives and midwives in the making. I'm honoured that you've chosen to prepare for your entry into midwifery with my book 'Becoming a Student Midwife'.

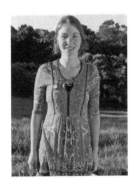

This book is full of information and advice gathered from midwives, midwifery interviewers, and careers advisers. It also puts together information from research papers, current understanding of psychology, university websites, forums and other sources. I've used this information along with my own experience of midwifery to offer the most comprehensive guide to the process I could muster.

Whether you're just at the beginning of your journey and are feeling passionate but overwhelmed and unsure how to start, or you've already been preparing for years and feel you just need to work out how to put all of your midwifery knowledge together, this guide can help. And now more than ever you'll need to be well armed when walking into your interview - I'll explain why below.

The focus of this book is to make you into the best applicant you can be. So if you believe you have what it takes to be a midwife, and you have something of real value to add to the profession, you will learn the techniques to get through the selection process and interview. You'll do this genuinely, without using 'stock phrases' or 'fooling' your interviewers - because the process is all about how best to present *your* unique personality and *your* unique talents within a midwifery context.

I wrote this book because midwifery is a career I care about and one crying out for the new clinicians, managers, researchers and specialists of the future. This book is helpful to the profession because it allows good candidates to shine and be identified, helping expand the talent of the profession.

It's common practice in other industries and jobs for candidates to refer to professional resources when preparing for interviews; it's high time midwives and prospective midwives had the opportunity to do the same!

That's what this book is all about: finding and giving a boost to midwives in the making.

I made it very difficult for myself when I was applying to be a midwife. In two terrible interviews I shook and stuttered, unsure of everything. It's so easy to become

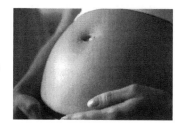

overwhelmed when you are interviewing for something you really care about.

But it's actually quite simple to prepare. Midwifery admissions tutors don't play games and they won't be trying to catch you out. You just have to master some basic skills like how to cope with your emotions, and how to see things from the point of view of a midwife, and learn a little about midwifery as a profession.

Once I worked out how to achieve these things, it all came quite naturally. I even started to enjoy interviews and I still do today - even though my initial gut feeling of 'flight or fight' hasn't changed! I want to help other people who would be excellent midwives learn how to do the application and interview process.

Why you need to be prepared

Getting onto a midwifery course has turned into a numbers game. Programmes like '*One Born Every Minute*' and '*Call The Midwife*' mean the world is waking up to the idea that midwifery is a job worth doing. The birth rate in the UK is rising, and partly because of this, many people are interested in helping out and training as midwives. However, at the same time the NHS is facing economic crisis, meaning that even though the UK is in desperate need of more midwives, funding for positions is limited.

This year's reports are of **one place for every 30-35 applicants** in universities. Often the competition is even tougher than that.

It's becoming monstrously competitive to get onto a course. It's not good enough to just do OK when 30 others might do the same. The techniques and inside knowledge in this book can help you become a midwife in the making with an edge. Doing this preparation will also help you see things from the point of view of a midwife, and therefore will actually make you into a better student midwife when you get your place on a course.

First, Check Midwifery Is Right For You

I'm not trying to put you off - I love supporting and empowering candidates. But I should let you know what you're letting yourself in for!

I would love to tell you that midwifery as a career is perfect. That you will glide into work at a reasonable time every morning with plenty of energy, spend endless meaningful hours with families, have lots of straightforward waterbirths and, in the evening, join your colleagues for a drink to discuss how wonderful your day was. But you already know better than that, and it's not the bargain we have struck.

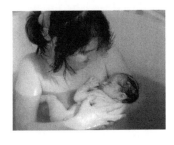

This is a life-changing path you are about to embark upon. Say 'midwife' and immediate connotations are of someone who is sympathetic, skilful, and mature. The responsibilities at times equal those of parenthood itself. The hours are long, unpredictable and full of tricky physiological assessments, difficult emotions and complex paperwork, often to be done in the wee hours, thirsty, hungry and full bladdered.

But that first listen in to a baby's heartbeat, empowering a scared mum or supporting a woman to give birth in her own way and watching the look on her face as she brings her baby up to her chest for the first time, are incomparably privileged experiences.

Helping someone becoming a good parent is so satisfying. It's a time of so much vulnerability and so much potential. I've lost count of how many times I've secretly cried after receiving heartfelt thanks to for good care, or I've been on an emotional high because a woman got the outcome she wanted. This is midwifery.

If all of that doesn't put you off, you may well have found your perfect career!

There are a few inside secrets I can share for this application process

Midwives and midwifery lecturers will be your interviewers. They are often impressive as they work on the 'shop floor' as midwives, while also lecturing, supporting students and may be undertaking postgraduate courses, juggling their responsibilities. However, they are nothing to be afraid of! This book will outline how to put yourself in their shoes and showcase yourself to them in the best possible light.

The book contains application notes, personal statement help and examples, effective advice on how to cope with nerves, basics like how to dress, how to approach group interview sessions, numeracy and literacy tests, presentations, and over 50 sample interview questions and answers. It has the essential tools to increase your confidence and will help you tackle difficult questions in your interview.

But most important of all, it will show you how to make yourself stand out as an impressive candidate who is remembered by the interviewers as the midwife in the making who shouldn't be passed up!

How To Get The Most Out Of This Book

If you are right at the beginning of your application, this book can be used as a guide to the whole process.

However, if you are part way through I have written the book so you can dip in and out of it easily. It's an inspirational application guide (with a sense of humour!). I personally find it helpful to highlight, underline and note down useful ideas or sentences that resonate with me in the margins.

- I am a learning book, write all over me! -

Free content, discussions and further advice is available on MidwifeDiaries.com. You can also come and get support from like-minded applicants and students at 'The Secret Community for Midwives in the Making' on Facebook. I'd love for you to get involved in the community.

As you work through the book, keep the following phrase in mind:

"Midwives in the making know it - but they also have to show it!"

In other words, you can have all the attributes and qualities of an excellent midwife, but if you can't show them to your admissions tutor, you won't get a place.

I wrote this book with this fact clearly in mind. As you read these chapters it's likely you will find you have most of what you need 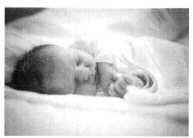 already – we just have to work out how to show the best of you…..

"Be yourself; everyone else is already taken."

--Oscar Wilde

"We are continually faced with great opportunities which are brilliantly disguised as unsolvable problems."

--Margaret Mead

Let's get going!

Chapter One: A Successful Application

Choosing Your University

The beginning of your journey - choosing where to train:

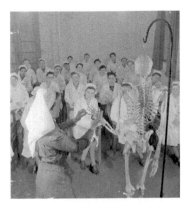

Choosing which universities to apply to can be a bit of a head scratch for prospective student midwives. Most students applying for degrees will look for the best universities for that subject; the ones with the best resources, reputation of getting their graduates jobs, and excellent lecturers - but midwifery doesn't work this way.

Midwifery is different because it's regulated. The Nursing and Midwifery Council makes sure all UK courses are of a standard that will train midwives to be competent practitioners. Therefore looking around online or in guides, it might appear there's not much to go on when choosing.

This can be a really good thing if you have family ties and can only apply to one or two universities as you can be sure of good training no matter where you end up. However, if you do have the luxury of choice, the following universities have an excellent reputation and are talked about well by student midwives on and offline (these are presented in no particular order):

• Southampton

• Nottingham

• Cardiff

• York

• Huddersfield

• Manchester

• De Montfort

As a De Montfort girl myself, I can say the course was excellent and had some wonderful midwife-teacher-author-researcher-lecturers!

• A good resource for further research, including a ranking system voted on by students, is the website whatuni.com.

Other Factors To Think About:

Where in the UK do you want to live? Would you prefer to be in London with lots going on?

Are you a walker who would love to be nearer the Peak District, so should consider Sheffield? Or are you a surfer who would love to be in Plymouth? All of these things will improve your experience and make it easier for you to find that mythical beast, a work/life balance. Ultimately this will help you train. It will also make it easier for you to say something positive about your choice of university at your interview.

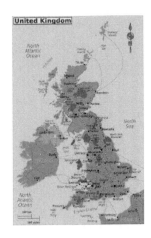

You should also consider what kind of midwife you are interested in becoming. Should you be somewhere which has a high homebirth rate and a few birth centres so you can get lots of low risk experience? Are you interested in rural placements? Or would you prefer somewhere like London for the hustle and bustle of a big city, lots of medical input and interesting socio-economic challenges? Knowing more about your prospective university will also help you write your personal statement and perform well in your interview.

It's also important to think about the nature of midwifery work; it's demanding, and there will be a lot of unsocial hours to put in. How close is your university to where you are going to live? Remember you will be coming home from placements at all hours, working 12 hour shifts overnight and perhaps on call. A short commute to university and placements will be greatly appreciated when you are tired.

You may want to look at what employment rates the universities have. Typically this is not because some universities produce great midwives and some don't - the number of midwives needed and the rate at which they move on from jobs is county specific. There is always a demand for more midwives in London, for instance, but in Scotland there is lower staff turnover so fewer people move around. This can also indicate better job satisfaction. Will you want to try somewhere new after your training, or would you prefer to have a greater chance of getting a job in your local area?

Thinking about who will support you during your training would also be a good idea. You may want to be close to your family, or a group of supportive friends. Midwifery is a very demanding course, and you might want to be able to get home within a short commute so someone can make you a cup of tea and give you a hug if you've had a challenging day!

If you can, go to university open days to help you decide. You can meet lecturers, talk to student midwives and ask lots of questions. It may all fall into place for you right there and then, and even if it doesn't, there are often lots of cool freebies!

Successfully Applying Through UCAS

Your application will go through UCAS (University College and Admissions Service), the government based organisation that sorts and sends applications.

Their website is easy to use, and you can always ring them for help. Make sure you type information clearly and accurately to create a good impression.

Universities may ask you to list other institutions you are applying to, either as part of your application or at an interview. I would politely decline, considering midwifery courses are oversubscribed and interviewers may be more likely to choose candidates who are just applying to their specific university - do not give away your cards if you don't have to.

References:

You will have to include two or more referees on your application. Obviously choose employers or teachers who will give you the best possible reference. If at all possible, brief them on mentioning your long passion for midwifery when talking to your chosen universities. A well-meaning referee mentioning that you have always wanted to be a nurse or do another course might mean your interviewer chooses someone else.

Entry Grades And How To Get Them

Specific UK midwifery entry requirements change frequently. Look at the university you are interested in to make sure. They will always have this information on their website. The bureaucracy involved in applying for different degree courses can vary greatly and will probably feel daunting at first. Be prepared to spend some time on it and it will be very achievable.

For example, within a few minutes I found the expected requirements for a midwifery degree at Manchester University in 2015, which were:

• 5 GCSEs at grade B or above to include Maths, English Language and a Science followed by:

• 3 A-levels at grades AAB or above, at least one to be in a science based subject like biology, physics, chemistry, sociology, psychology, etc. or equivalent grades in an applicable BTEC or another applicable route (further information is available on their website)

If you don't have the required qualifications:

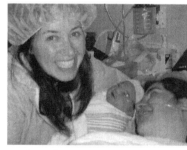

There are various 'Access to Higher Education' ('Access to HE') courses available either as distance learning courses or at village or city colleges. Going to the 'Access to Higher Education' website (www.accesstohe.ac.uk) will put you on the right track.

To undertake an Access to HE course you will usually need GCSEs (or equivalent) in English, Maths and Science at grade C or above. If you need GCSEs or need to improve your grades, the National Extension

College is a good distance learning provider (www.nec.ac.uk/). Funding is often available.

However, if you believe you have enough academic, professional and life experience to train as a midwife, it's well worth putting in a strong application even if you fall short of the qualifications.

I would ring up and talk to the Head of Department and explain exactly why you think you meet the requirements. Do this with a confident but not arrogant attitude. **I can't guarantee you'll be offered an interview, but interviewers do value character and experience.** The worst that will happen is you will be refused with more idea of what is required from you for the next year; the best will be you get an interview. The interviewers will also know you, and your commitment at trying again next year will be to your advantage.

Getting Experience and Volunteering

If you're serious about getting a place on a midwifery course, you **need** some practical experience! I can't stress enough how crucial this is. For interviewers, this is often the most important demonstration of your commitment and suitability. Midwives tend to value experience above all else, as they work in practical situations and are used to holding in high esteem any of their staff who can just 'get on with it'!

You can ring or email your local hospital and ask to volunteer specifically on a maternity ward. If you are put through 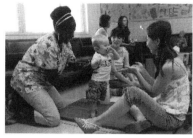 to labour ward or another maternity ward be aware it can be so busy the staff might not have had a break for the last 8 or even 12 hours - keep your request brief and polite and don't be offended if they refuse! If they do let you volunteer, you've hit the jackpot.

If not, be **resourceful**. Anyone should be able to get a bit of specific experience, but don't worry if it's not attending births as this is not essential. In fact a lot of midwives will say 'anyone can catch a baby, it's everything else that's important'. Some of these options are very time effective, yet prove your commitment and suitability.

Choose at least one of the following:

• Use a social media tool to search for midwives you can take out for coffee to discuss what their job is like; make notes on the interview (*no, I'm not just hoping to be taken out for a coffee!*)

• La Leche League breastfeeding support groups are found in most areas; ask to go along to a 'breastfeeding cafe' and help out.

• Call the National Childbirth Trust and ask for permission to call some women who use their services - put together some questions for them and listen to 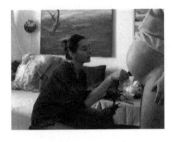 their impressions of NHS maternity care.

• Ask to attend or help with local parentcraft classes.

• Research independent midwives online and ask to shadow one for a day.

• Work as a healthcare assistant in a ward or care home. I would combine this option with one of the other midwifery specific options.

• Perhaps look into getting some midwifery experience abroad. You may be able to do something really useful and beneficial for a community at the same time as getting experience, travelling, and adding interest to your application! You will however have to be careful to do an ethical volunteer placement in which you will gain some midwifery experience (as some developing countries have little legal protection about care and how qualified you have to be to get involved).

Whatever experience you get, keep **records** of your thoughts, who you met, what skills you developed or knowledge you gained, and how it all relates back to your goal of being a midwife.

Remember to keep any clients anonymous and untraceable in your notes as this is essential to show you can handle confidential information. This is one area I would be very careful about as a lack of discretion could put your place at risk.

Computer And Research Tricks

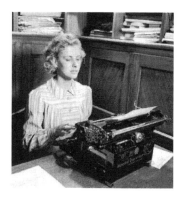

If you already use computers without issues you can skip this section if you like...however there are some tricks I'd learnt by the end of my training which would have knocked hours off researching and finding information over the course of my degree! I wish I'd known this stuff before I started applying to be a student midwife.

This is essentially a cheat's guide to researching, combined with a few computer life hacks for midwives. I'm genuinely surprised that even some very tech savvy people I'm friends with don't know this stuff!

• A good old Google search can serve you well even when looking at an academic topic; don't underestimate it.

• Google Scholar is a search engine for academic resources including lots of research papers and journals - just remember, you have to be able to tell which research studies are good ones. The odds are that if they've been quoted positively by official organisations like the Royal College of Midwives or Royal College of Obstetricians and Gynaecologists, they will be reliable.

• Many search engines have a 'discussion' search tool which finds forum discussions. This is useful, as the odds are that someone, somewhere has already received answers in reply to a question similar to yours. Type your search term into the search engine's search bar, for instance 'waterbirth', and add the word 'discussion' at the end.

• There's nothing wrong with **skim reading** and just focussing on particular paragraphs; academic performance is all about the ability to take in information quickly and filtering out the irrelevant stuff.

• Blogs and websites such as MidwifeDiaries.com; Sarawickham.com, Gasandairblog.com, Midwifethinking.com, Evidencebasedbirth.com and others can offer significant insight into different topics.

• Google Books has many previews of textbooks and other materials to do with midwifery.

Some of my colleagues seem to think Wikipedia, the online encyclopaedia, is the spawn of all misinformation. It's written by unpaid anonymous internet users. However it attracts expert authors, and **articles are evidence based and up to date.** 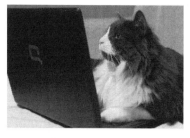 There is competitive pride around writing a good Wikipedia article that makes it a good resource.

Because Wikipedia is visited so many times a day by so many people, inaccuracy or vandalism is picked up lightning fast. Crucially, **the information on Wikipedia can be checked for authenticity** by following the links to source material at the bottom and it's in this way I use it to guide my practice or to write essays. You can use it to research midwifery topics all the way through your application process.

And the most important tool of all, which astonishingly few people seem to know about: You can search and jump to any word/phrase in any article or document by simultaneously holding down the **control 'Ctrl' + f** keys, and then typing in the word you want to find on your current page or document.

'Control' + 'f' will bring up a search bar which will find your word and allow you to jump through multiple instances of it in the page or document.

For instance, if I am on the Royal College of Midwives site, and I want to see if there are any mentions of interviews on the page, I simply hold 'control + f' and a search bar will appear, usually in the top right of the screen. I can type 'interview', and jump through entries of this word.

This works for any document or webpage (or email or article for that matter). It will stop you from having to wade through literally hundreds of thousands of irrelevant words!

This shortcut also work on Mac computers; just use the 'Command' key instead of 'Control'.

Chapter Two: Your Personal Statement

Introduction

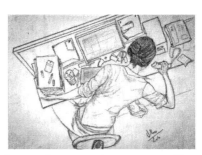

Your personal statement is your time to shine! It is your most important persuasive tactic to get an interview and it's **worth preparing very well**. A professionally written and engaging statement will help get you to the interview stage, but it will also prime your interviewers to expect an impressive candidate on interview day. It can be your ticket to getting onto a midwifery course.

Applying for midwifery means writing a **targeted personal statement**. It has to be **all about midwifery**. A statement that shows you are interested in both midwifery and another choice, for instance nursing, might well cause your rejection. This is because midwifery is very oversubscribed and it's like no other career on earth!

If you do want nursing or another course as your backup in order to start training as soon as possible, I still suggest applying for midwifery using all five of your choices. If you are unsuccessful, you can reapply to do nursing or another course using UCAS Extra.

This service helps you apply to further universities after the cut-off date (usually 30th June), and you can find more details at:

www.ucas.com/how-it-all-works/undergraduate/tracking-your-application/adding-extra-choices

You will be able to resubmit an alternate personal statement; nursing and most other courses are not oversubscribed in the same way as midwifery, and you have a much higher chance of getting a place if you do things this way. **It's all about using the UCAS system to your advantage!**

The Basics

You will be able to find dates for submission of applications on the UCAS website. Usually applications open in mid- 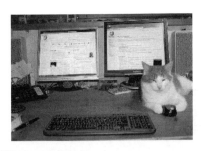 September, and cut off by mid-January.

You are best off applying as soon as possible. Midwifery admissions tutors look at applications chronologically, as they come in, meaning you stand a better chance if you're early rather than late.

There are a few major rules I recommend sticking to when writing your personal statement:

• Be formal. Slang or informal language is best avoided as the admissions tutors are trying to work out if you can be professional.

• Be yourself! Don't feel like you have to use complex language. Be polite and aim for a professional tone, but try and let your personality come across too. It's better to use language you are familiar with, for instance 'It feels like a career I would be good at' as opposed to 'Midwifery is my 'raison d'être' '.

• Keep it simple. **Your admissions tutors will be busy people, just like you.** Make your points clearly: for instance instead of saying, 'Hiking has taught me how to orienteer, and this will help in midwifery because of the transferable skills of resilience and keeping calm', try 'Hiking has taught me to keep a clear head under stress, even when lost. I imagine this is the attitude needed on a midwifery ward when it's very busy or when there is an emergency.'

• Make sure your spelling and grammar are perfect!

• Avoid acronyms and abbreviations, for instance use 'and so on' instead of 'etc'.

• Use all the characters available and avoid repetition.

• Concentrate on the positive aspects of your application. The admissions tutors will have no problem identifying your weaknesses. Mentioning or trying to explain them in your personal statement will not be expected and consequently may make you seem under confident.

• Have structure: your admissions tutors will usually only have around 15 minutes to look at each statement. Therefore your statement needs to flow, to help the admissions tutors navigate through your skills and experience.

There is no one right way to structure a personal statement. However, if you would like to use a pre-determined structure, the following is a tried and tested method:

1. An introduction, describing why you want to be a midwife, or that shows a fascinating, individual experience or insight you have.
2. A brief description of your academic background and discussion of how you will cope with the theory component of the course, including time management skills (most of this information will be on your application so this section should be short).
3. A discussion of your shadowing/volunteer/work experience, and the transferrable skills you gained. Demonstrate your understanding of midwifery.
4. Any life experience which might have important transferrable skills.
5. Your personal take on midwifery.
6. A conclusion which sums up why you are an excellent candidate.

You may want to have a **specialist interest subject** that you can draw on throughout your personal statement. This subject should be close to your heart or interests, and you should research it really thoroughly.

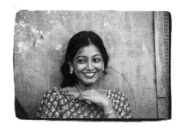

It's a bit hard to explain why having a specialist interest subject you know a lot about will help you so much. But whether you're new to midwifery as a subject, or you have lots of knowledge already, in so many ways it will add **depth and focus to your statement, application and interview.** You will see why and how as you continue through the book, especially in Chapter Five: *"Above and Beyond"*.

You should choose a topic you find fascinating. Some ideas include:

• The impact of poverty on midwifery outcomes

• Teenage pregnancy

• Ethnic minorities and language barriers

• Obesity

• Waterbirth

• Mental Illness

There is a good 'personal statement calculator' at www.maccery.com/ps/. UCAS uses a character rather than a word count - this means it counts letters, numbers, symbols, spaces and any time you choose to make a new line. Either cut and paste your 4000 character personal statement into the tool or type it in if you have written it by hand. It will show you any formatting issues.

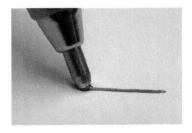

There are three personal statements in this chapter. Each personal statement is followed by an analysis that identifies the good techniques and mistakes.

This chapter purposefully doesn't have a template or 'formula' for you to follow. It's truly about educating yourself to write well. Using the techniques in this chapter will help you come across as an exceptional candidate, without using **clichéd phrases or ideas,** an **over confident tone** or **ubiquitous content.**

It can be really hard to even start writing a personal statement as most of us are not used to blowing our own trumpets! It's a lot of pressure to be under, and it's easy to feel like you're writing a load of cobblers.

But try not to fall into the trap of believing you have to write a perfect personal statement as soon as you get typing. Just get some ideas down, mind maps can be a very good starting point. You'll be able to edit it into something really impressive - it can even be fun! Imagine the admissions tutors reading a personal statement that will make them really excited about an excellent midwife in the making!

The first example statement is riddled with common errors candidates make.

Be smart and avoid these mistakes - this knowledge has come from university admissions tutors, professional careers advisers, the Royal College of Midwives and my own personal experience in helping candidates edit and perfect their personal statements. Try and spot the errors as you read through and I'll tell you what the admissions tutor will be thinking in the analysis section.

Personal Statement Example 1: Common Mistakes

Since my sister had my Niece three years ago I have been obsessed with the beauty of birth. Though I have not been pregnant myself I believe our closeness gave me real insight into what it's like to be pregnant and give birth. I also love babies. Because of this I think I would make an excellent nurse or midwife.

I believe I would make an excellent midwife based on my experience with my niece and the fact I am a kind and compassionate person. I have not had children myself yet (I can't convince my boyfriend!) so I feel my maternal instincts would be put to better use elsewhere.

I feel that my A-level choices, which I chose specifically to become a midwife are very good. Chemistry covers medications and an understanding of the basics of science. I believe studying French has opened my mind to another culture which is an important skill. My final subject Drama and Theatre Studies I believe allows me to communicate better and work in teams, both key skills for midwives.

Although I haven't quite made the grades in my mock exams, I want to be a midwive so much I know when the real exam period comes along I will find the answers somehow, even though I am very busy! My teachers all say I am very hardworking and that I should definitely work in a caring profession. I am always the class member who students come to when they want advice.

In terms of experience I have worked for a few days in a carehome with the elderly. I know this doesn't apply directly to midwifery but it is difficult to find experience where I live. Additionally as I mentioned above I have good personal experience helping care for a pregnant women and a baby who are close to me personally.

I have done lots of reading on midwifediaries.com and also from journals such as NZCOM, Journal of Midwifery and Women's Health, and done a lot of reading of NCT leaflets. I am a big fan of breastfeeding based on this reading. I've watched every episode of One Born Every Minute, I know all the patients' stories and names of their babies. I also know all about the Nursing Council and the way midwives have to take their lead from them.

I would of course personally breastfeed and encourage women of all ages and backgrounds to take on this fantastic privilege. I would work hard to make sure none of my patients wanted to bottlefeed their babies.

Midwifery is my dream job because of the amazing relationships I will make with the women and my colleagues. I believe to be a midwife you must be an incredible, understanding person and therefore I look forward to learning so much around teachers and midwives. I read a quote online recently that a midwife must have the hands of a lady, the eyes of a hawk and the heart of a lion. I believe I am indeed gentle, observant and very brave. I am not at all squeamish at the sight of blood. Although I think nightshifts and working weekends would be very difficult as I have a very busy social life and a large circle of friends, I am good at staying up at night and my motivation is so great I could work through this.

I am fit and healthy and like dancing, reading midwifery texts and in my spare time I like to watch videos on YouTube. I do hope you will consider my application strongly as I have only applied for nursing as my other university option but I would much prefer midwifery. Although Kings College London would be my top choice I would be happy at the other places I have applied to. God Bless and thankyou for your time.

Personal Statement Example 1: Analysis

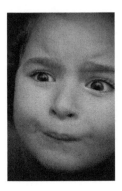

I'm sure you picked up on some of the problems in this statement!

The first thing to note about this personal statement is that it is 250 or so characters too short. You should aim to fill all the space you are given as you have precious little to demonstrate how impressive you are.

"Since my sister had my Niece three years ago I have been obsessed with the beauty of birth. Though I have not been pregnant myself I believe our closeness gave me real insight into what it's like to be pregnant and give birth. Because of this I think I would make an excellent nurse or midwife."

Be careful about using personal experience as a justification for becoming a midwife. Although having a baby or being close to someone having a baby is often an excellent start to your interest, heartfelt emotions are not always what is needed when working as a midwife in 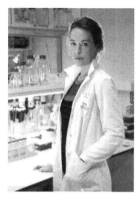 a busy area. **Objectivity along with passion for birth** is perhaps closer to what you want to get across. This candidate has also mentioned nursing - this will indicate to the admissions tutors that she is not that serious about midwifery.

"I also love babies."

This is a really common mistake listed by universities and the Royal College of Midwives. It is very positive this candidate wants to work with babies but the word midwife literally means **'with women'** and that's what's the job is about. The admissions tutors will be thinking, why doesn't she want to be a nursery nurse, or a neonatal nurse, or a paediatrician if she loves babies so much? Try and make the majority of what you say **midwifery focussed**, talk about the women.

"I believe I would make an excellent midwife based on my experience with my niece and the fact I am a kind and compassionate person. I have not had children myself yet (I can't convince my boyfriend!) so I feel my

maternal instincts would be put to better use elsewhere."

Being kind and compassionate are good qualities, but demonstrating how these qualities impact positively on the role of a midwife would have been better. Humour is almost certainly not a good idea unless you have an exceptional point to make and you are extremely confident it will not be misinterpreted. Additionally, while your maternal or paternal instincts may be of use at times as a midwife, it's not something your admissions tutors will be looking for, and too much of it will be off-putting.

"I feel that my A-level choices, which I chose specifically to be able to apply to become a midwife, are very good. Chemistry covers medications and an understanding of the basics of science. I believe studying French has opened my mind to another culture which is an important skill. My final subject Drama and Theatre Studies I believe allows me to communicate better and work in teams, both key skills for midwives."

Do not put anything that could interpreted as a lie on your personal statement. Claiming A-level choices of Chemistry, French and Drama were chosen specifically to support entry to midwifery doesn't sound very realistic. Why didn't this candidate choose biology, sociology, women's studies, perhaps philosophy, ethics or an access to midwifery course? It's fine to justify your A-levels and the transferable skills they have. You may even show the admissions tutors you are an interesting 'find' if you have not taken a traditional route. But what you write has to be realistic, and in this instance it's not.

"Although I haven't quite made the grades in my mock exams, I want to be a midwive so much I know when the real exam period comes along I will find the answers somehow, even though I am very busy!"

Misspelling midwife or midwives will almost certainly mean you are rejected as it shows you haven't taken much care. Decide whether your statement will have the profession capitalised ('Midwife', 'Midwives', 'Midwifery') or lower case ('midwife', 'midwives', 'midwifery') and stick to it to show consistency. Getting your personal statement proof read by a professional such as a teacher or someone at a free job advice centre will definitely help with this, especially if you suffer from dyslexia or another writing problem. It's worth submitting something with perfect spelling and grammar - these are easy things to get right even if you have to get professional help!

As an aside: if you are dyslexic or have another learning difficulty, don't for a moment think you won't be a good midwife. Many very competent midwives I have worked with have had learning disabilities and were well supported by, as well as being supportive to, their colleagues.

Avoid making any references to negative aspects of your application, be it academic or otherwise, as our candidate has done here. The admissions tutors won't have any trouble identifying your weaknesses and you won't be expected to talk about them in your personal statement.

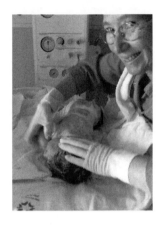

The candidate in this case might have been better off stressing good organisational skills instead of telling the admissions tutors about her busy schedule. **A very important point to realise is that your admissions tutors are likely to be midwives who are incredibly busy themselves.** As mentioned in the introduction to this book, some of my admissions tutors were PhD students, worked part time on the 'shop floor' of labour or other maternity wards, lectured and supported students and interviewed for new candidates, and some will have young children on top of all that!

"My teachers all say I am very hardworking and that I should definitely work in a caring profession. I am always the class member who students come to when they want advice."

Show, don't tell; this candidate has merely stated what her teachers think of her. It's far better to demonstrate exactly why you are hardworking and would be good in a caring profession. Do you work extra hours in a care home around your college studies? Do you find this is the most rewarding part of your week? These are good examples of your suitability.

Try to present your **active listening** skills as well as your advising skills as these will be needed most as a new student midwife.

"In terms of experience I have worked in a carehome with the elderly. I know this doesn't apply directly to midwifery but it is difficult to find experience where I live. Additionally as I mentioned above I have good personal experience helping care for a pregnant women and a newborn who are close to me personally."

Again, the general rule with personal statements is to frame everything in a positive light. This candidate could have talked about becoming more compassionate, more able to understand the needs of bed-bound people, and aware of the need to inspire confidence so people can feel well. Also, don't come up with excuses if you feel something is lacking. Enthuse about the experience you have.

This candidate has also mentioned her niece numerous times. With the character limit imposed by UCAS you need to avoid repetition, both to give yourself more space to show how brilliant you are, and to avoid seeming disorganised.

"I have done lots of reading on midwifediaries.com and also from journals such as NZCOM, Journal of Midwifery and Women's Health, and done a lot of reading of NCT leaflets."

Academic reading is excellent and it's great to include a few lines on interesting research you've come across. However, admissions tutors might be less enthusiastic about forums or websites. This is a formal introduction to you, and mentioning a recently published peer reviewed journal article (from the Lancet, British Journal of Midwifery or somewhere similar) would be more impressive.

This candidate has also rather strangely mentioned the NZCOM (the New Zealand College of Midwives) journal without justifying why she has chosen research conducted 12,000 miles away from her prospective workplace. Her admissions tutors might be thinking, 'Why not a British journal, so this candidate can get educated about at-home matters before looking at midwifery globally?' There are very good reasons to look at research journals from New Zealand, but this candidate needs to mention what they are!

NCT (National Childbirth Trust) leaflets are also mentioned, but these are for clients and are possibly not detailed enough for someone wanting to be a healthcare professional.

Mentioning you like to read up to date journals on midwifery research and then sharing a detailed factual analysis of what you found would be much more striking.

"I am a big fan of breastfeeding based on this reading."

Breastfeeding has been a controversial topic within midwifery for a long time, and is brilliant to discuss in a personal statement. However it's best not to come across as too militant in your approach to breastfeeding - promoting and supporting it is great, coercing isn't.

This candidate has also split her views on breastfeeding between this sentence and a paragraph further down. It is better to have a good structure to your personal statement based on the 'point - example - explain' model of writing unless there is an exceptional point to make that benefits from being split.

"I've watched every episode of One Born Every Minute, I know all the patients' stories and names of their babies."

Watching 'One Born Every Minute' is something a lot of TV watchers do and does not demonstrate a good understanding of midwifery, at least on its own. From the

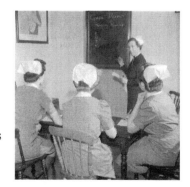

admissions tutors' point of view, watching every episode may be time better spent getting experience or reading factual information.

"I also know all about the Nursing Council and the way midwives have to take their lead from them."

Every year candidates makes this mistake: they either write or imply midwifery is similar to nursing. In fact **nursing and midwifery are very different.** Midwifery philosophy is based around the premise of caring for well women and babies. Nursing is defined by caring for unwell people. If you compare midwifery to nursing in your statement, you're showing lack of insight.

Midwives have had a long legal battle to regain their autonomy from nursing and other medical professions. Midwives are regulated by the Nursing and Midwifery Council - not the 'Nursing Council' - and midwives certainly do not take their lead from them! I can imagine a few of my more passionate colleagues getting quite cross at this sentence.

For more information on the Nursing and Midwifery Council, see Chapter Four, page 85.

"I would of course personally breastfeed and encourage women of all ages and backgrounds to take on this fantastic privilege. I would work hard to make sure none of my patients wanted to bottlefeed their babies."

As I mentioned above, **midwives do not force their clients into decisions**. This candidate might appear over-enthusiastic, perhaps even controlling when it comes to breastfeeding.

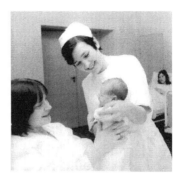

Acknowledging that breastfeeding support is a challenge, but one that is exciting, might be better. There is a chance that the bit about the candidate 'personally breastfeeding' could also be interpreted as meaning that the candidate plans to personally breastfeed babies in her care, which is a bit worrying!

Referring to women as 'patients' is not the best choice of words. Midwifery philosophy aims for normal, physiological childbearing; 'clients' or simply 'women' may be better choices.

"Midwifery is my dream job because of the amazing relationships I will make with the women and my colleagues. I believe to be a midwife you must be an incredible, understanding person and therefore I look forward to learning so much around teachers and midwives."

The passionate nature of this paragraph is good. However the candidate does not demonstrate she understands the challenges of training. Your admissions tutors will be acutely that the pressures of the job means learning can be full of criticism, high pressure situations and brisk explanations. I would emphasise instead how much you're looking forward to the challenge of working in a busy midwifery environment and learning from midwives with lots of experience.

"I read a quote online recently that a midwife must have the hands of a lady, the eyes of a hawk and the heart of a lion. I believe I am indeed gentle, observant and very brave. I am not at all squeamish at the sight of blood."

Quotes are tricky to use in personal statements. I have anecdotal evidence that some admissions tutors don't favour them. They are often more trouble than they're worth because they don't say enough about you as an individual.

However, there is nothing wrong with including a quote that makes an excellent point. Sometimes someone else has put your thoughts into words so brilliantly that you'd be reinventing the wheel by trying to rewrite them. But choose with care, know exactly the reason you are putting your quote in - what brilliant and individual point does it make about you?

This historic quote from Aristotle does illustrate some of the key qualities a midwife needs - but in some admissions tutors' eyes, it might be quite superficial in a modern midwifery context. You should also include quotation marks if you use a quote.

Also, this candidate's ability to deal with body fluids might well be already assumed as she is applying to train as a midwife. It's not necessary to mention this in your statement.

"Although I think nightshifts and working weekends would be very difficult as I have a very busy social life and a large circle of friends, I am good at staying up at night and my motivation is so great I could work through this."

Again, this candidate would do better to avoid mentioning negative aspects of midwifery. Put a positive light on things. Mentioning how well you will cope with shiftwork is a good idea (as long as it's true). Prior experience with shiftwork or suggesting a good coping 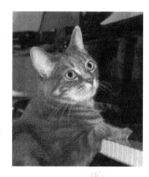 mechanism, for instance a supportive partner, is what they will be looking for.

Mentioning you have a very busy social life may be reassuring in some ways for your admissions tutors as they will be able to see you are a people person. However, midwifery is very time consuming, and admissions tutors will be concerned if you hint at an already packed schedule.

"I am fit and healthy and like dancing, reading midwifery texts and in my spare time I like to watch videos on YouTube."

Mentioning you are fit and healthy is a good idea as midwifery is a physical job.

Mentioning your hobbies and interests is an excellent idea to show a good attitude to work/life balance. For this reason in this section I would avoid mentioning midwifery related activities. Try to include your most commendable hobby - watching YouTube videos is something most people do, and besides, your admissions tutors will probably struggle to find many transferrable skills that can be gained from watching videos of piano-playing cats!

"I do hope you will consider my application strongly as I have only applied for nursing as my other university option but I would much prefer midwifery. Although Kings College London would be my top choice I would be happy at the other places I have applied to."

Again, this candidate has referred to nursing and this will count against her.

As UCAS do not allow students to write more than one personal statement you should not mention any universities specifically, especially not to prioritise one above others as the admissions tutors may find this unimpressive!

If you are applying for one university only, read the 'Research your University' section in Chapter Four, page 90. Use the tips on giving an outstanding interview to write a targeted personal statement. It's also a good idea to mention you really want to go to that particular university in your statements for extra brownie points.

"God Bless and thank you for your time."

'God Bless' suggests a religious belief. As a midwife you will have to look after women from many cultures and belief systems. If you mention you are religious it might be best to explain how well you will cope with the differences between your and your clients' beliefs. Mentioning you are an active member at your local place of worship may be a tactful way of explaining your beliefs, but outlining your beliefs or mentioning you think midwifery is in part a religious calling for you may be misguided.

The next statement features excellent techniques and strategies all the way through. Try to work out what they are and then find out more ways to present yourself as a brilliant midwife in the making in the analysis section.

Personal Statement Example 2: Excellent Technique

Midwifery for me represents the best type of modern holistic healthcare. It's a testament to how far society has come that medicine and maternity care can work in partnership with women.

I have worked to get the high grades necessary to study as a student midwife. I am passionate about my A-

level subjects; Biology, Chemistry and Classical Civilisations. The transferrable skills/knowledge from the first two qualifications are beneficial in terms of physiology, studying pharmacology, and so on, but you may well ask why I chose Classics. It was because I believe you should study what you find fascinating, even though I initially didn't see the connection to midwifery. However, Classics provided me with an understanding of how modern medicine developed. It also made me appreciate the role of women as key players in history both on their own account and because of their childbearing. This knowledge helped me to re-appreciate the impact of midwives as facilitators of healthy mothers and newborns, and their effect on society.

I understand it must be easy to see midwifery through 'rose tinted glasses', so I volunteered at the National Childbirth Trust parentcraft organisation. This was beneficial not only because of the basic knowledge about childbearing I developed but also because women told stories of their babies being born, naturally, assisted or via caesarean. This helped me to appreciate the responsibilities a midwife must face in terms of expectations in a busy and economically challenged NHS. I understand a midwife's role must be very challenging in terms of the different support s/he must offer, be it for medical care, natural childbirth, supporting grief or working with social issues. I would have loved the opportunity to work in a maternity unit, but instead I volunteered in an elderly ward, which gave me an understanding of the way hospitals are run. I was able to learn how to do basic observations, bed changes, cares, and providing just 'someone to talk to'. Talking to qualified midwives, the ability to quickly form a relationship and help clients with intimate care is an essential transferable skill I developed.

I have enjoyed reading academic texts and journals on midwifery, in particular some of Soo Downe et al's most recent work on the routine use of vaginal examinations during normal labour (2013). I have a particular interest in the impact of culture and personalities on midwifery care, and although I wouldn't dream of applying this kind of research without experience and guidance, it is interesting to see the progress of midwifery care and its influences, not all of which are evidence based. In terms of texts I have found Ina May Gaskin's 'Spiritual Midwifery' very useful to give a flavour of the political changes around birth, but also because of the way she prioritises the individualised relationship of respect between midwife and client. Her simple notes on the physiology and mechanism of childbirth are also very interesting.

I have always been a hard worker but I do think balance is essential, and I enjoy life! My long term boyfriend is very supportive and we enjoy going fishing and walking. I have a good circle of friends who enjoy live music and karaoke. I love being physically active and I think this helps with motivation and feeling well. My friends think it's funny that I'm so interested in midwifery at an early age, but they are very supportive and think it's a career that fits my personality. I have given thought to the long hours and shift work involved and feel I have the skills necessary to achieve a good work/life balance long term, based on the time I spent on the ward.

I understand midwifery is a career which many people want to join. I'd like to finish by saying that all I can bring you is a passion for the subject, motivation, a keen interest in the way midwifery care changes based on society and an appreciation of how much impact the professional relationship between midwife and women can have.

Personal Statement Example 2: Analysis

At three characters under the maximum, this candidate has obviously taken time to craft her personal statement. It is well balanced, and covers her academic, practical, and personal suitability to train as a midwife.

"Midwifery for me represents the best type of modern holistic healthcare. It's a testament to how far society has come that medicine and maternity care can work in partnership with women."

The opening statement covers an interesting and complex opinion about midwifery and why it's such an exciting profession. By having this opinion the candidate is **showing** instead of telling her enthusiasm and understanding for midwifery.

Remember: *"Midwives in the making know it - but they also have to show it!"*

"I have worked to get the high grades necessary to study as a student midwife. I am passionate about my A-level subjects; Biology, Chemistry and Classical Civilisations. The transferrable skills/knowledge from the first two qualifications are beneficial in terms of physiology, studying pharmacology and so on but you may well ask why I chose Classics. It was because I believe you should study what you find fascinating, even though I initially didn't see the connection to midwifery. However Classics provided me with an understanding of how modern medicine developed. It also made me appreciate the role of women as key players in history both on their own account and because of their childbearing. This knowledge helped

me to re-appreciate the impact of midwives as facilitators of healthy mothers and newborns, and their effect on society."

This candidate has chosen two subjects applicable to midwifery but one subject, Classics, is a bit more of a stretch. Identifying briefly why Biology and Chemistry are useful in the profession shows an appreciation of the role of a midwife, but analysing Classics for its usefulness makes this candidate **memorable and shows she can think for herself.**

The bit about 'studying what you find fascinating' is good, because it shows **enthusiasm for academic work.** The admissions tutors know you will need to juggle a heavy schedule with essays and exams, so will try and work out how you're likely to cope from your statement.

The point made about midwifery care in a historical context also shows the ability to think academically, and is interesting and well described.

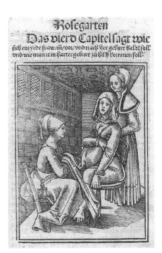

It's worth mentioning however that you will be expected to be able to talk about any point made in your personal statement, so

don't write anything you wouldn't be happy to be quizzed about!

It is also easy if you're in the middle of your A-levels or equivalent to write too much about academic ability. Midwifery is a practical skill, and luckily this candidate moves onto her experience in the next paragraph. Any more discussion of her college career might make the admissions tutors think she is only interested in midwifery in an academic way.

"I understand it must be easy to see midwifery through 'rose tinted glasses', so I volunteered at the National Childbirth Trust parentcraft organisation. This was beneficial not only because of the basic knowledge about childbearing I developed, but also because women told stories of their babies being born, naturally, assisted or via caesarean. This helped me to appreciate the responsibilities a midwife must face in terms of expectations in a busy and economically challenged NHS. I understand a midwife's role must be very challenging in terms of the different support s/he must offer, be it medical care, natural childbirth, supporting grief or working with social issues."

Having an unrealistic or undeveloped view of midwifery is a common reason admissions tutors refuse applicants. This candidate has gone out of her way to find out what is really expected of midwives. Although attending National Childbirth Trust classes is something almost anyone can do, she has extracted a lot from the experience. She shows her active listening skills by supporting women telling their stories. She has also noted the economic strain that midwives face which shows her up to date understanding.

Admissions tutors will be looking for a broad understanding of the role of a midwife. The last sentence of this paragraph touches neatly on the spectrum of care, and tactfully on grief and social issues. These topics are massively challenging areas of midwifery care. Many candidates don't know how to talk about grief from unexpected outcomes, deaths or social issues like alcoholism, drug abuse and violence. Although focussing on these issues in too much depth in your personal statement may seem morbid, if you don't mention them at all the admissions tutors might think that you don't understand the sad or distressing aspects of midwifery.

"I would have loved the opportunity to work in a maternity unit, but instead I volunteered in an elderly ward, which gave me an understanding of the way hospitals are run. I was able to learn how to do basic observations, bed changes, cares, and providing just 'someone to talk to'."

This candidate has not been able to get experience shadowing a midwife or on a labour ward, but they have tried to get some applicable skills. This shows determination. A basic understanding of the way wards are run is very valuable. Being able to do observations like blood pressure, temperature and pulse are also brilliant skills to have. A willingness to help with intimate care also **shows rather than tells** suitability and a lack of squeamishness.

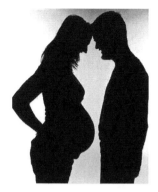

"Talking to qualified midwives, the ability to quickly form a relationship and help clients with intimate care is an essential transferable skill I developed."

This is an excellent observation, as it's a central skill! Midwifery at its heart is all about being personable and gaining the trust of the clients in your care. It tells the admissions tutors this candidate has insight.

"I have enjoyed reading academic texts and journals on midwifery, in particular some of Soo Downe et al's most recent work on the 'Routine use of vaginal examinations during normal labour' (2013). I have a particular interest in the impact of culture and personality on midwifery care. Although I wouldn't dream of applying this kind of research without experience and guidance, it is interesting to see the

progress of midwifery care and its influences, not all of which are evidence based."

This candidate has chosen a well-known and well regarded researcher to read, showing she is on the right 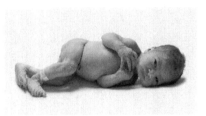 track in her exploration of the subject. She might know that Soo Downe has written many contemporary books on midwifery that are on most university midwifery degree reading lists.

The candidate has provided a year (2013) for the piece of research, which hints at her ability to write academically. It is also a cutting edge piece of research published in the same year she is applying. She has chosen a specific topic she has interest for, i.e. cultural and personal influences on midwifery. As discussed above, this makes her memorable and provides some depth to her statement.

Examining research tactfully without attacking midwives is beneficial. The piece of research looks at whether or not women are examined for good reasons in labour. If the candidate had enthused about her ability to change an aspect of midwifery she may have been seen by the admissions tutors as getting a bit ahead of herself.

It's best not to criticise current practice at this point. You can suggest changes need to be made, but there's a fine line between confidence and arrogance.

"In terms of texts I have found Ina May Gaskin's 'Spiritual Midwifery' very useful to give a flavour of the political changes around birth, but also because of the way she prioritises the individualised relationship of respect between midwife and client. Her simple notes on the physiology and mechanism of childbirth are also very interesting."

Ina May Gaskin is a well-known controversial figure in midwifery. She and her team of self-taught midwives (they do not pursue a certified training route) have exceptionally good outcomes, but some argue her low key attitude to complex childbirth situations deserves scrutiny, and that her statistics may be skewed.

This candidate has shown she is aware of the political situation around birth, represented by Ina May Gaskin. She has quite cleverly chosen an aspect of her style of care that can't be argued with: her prioritisation of the personal relationship between midwife and woman. This is a safe way to show the depth and breadth of your reading. There is a lot of time to debate about the politics around childbirth when you are on the course, but it will be expected that your personal statement 'plays it safe'.

This candidate has also commented on her interest of the 'physiology and mechanism of childbirth', which is music to any lecturer's ears!

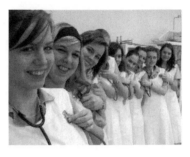

"I have always been a hard worker, but I do think balance is essential and I enjoy life! My long term boyfriend is very supportive and we enjoy going fishing and walking. I have a good circle of friends who enjoy live music and karaoke, and I love being physically active and think this helps with motivation and feeling well."

Showing a good work/life balance is essential within your personal statement. It shows emotional stability, interpersonal skills, and your ability to cope with a demanding course without 'burning out'. Being physically active is also very important, as midwifery is a demanding job with a fair amount of contorting into strange positions to catch babies and help with breastfeeding! Many midwives have had to retire or give up because of back problems.

"My friends think it's funny that I'm so interested in midwifery at an early age, but they are very supportive and think it's a career that fits my personality."

If you are age 17-20 and have recently left full time education (as I had when applying!), it may be best to put in a sentence acknowledging it is a big career decision to take at a young age. It doesn't have to be explicit or excuse your age. As I mentioned before, it's best not to identify your weaknesses in your personal statement and this still holds true.

But a few midwifery admissions tutors I can think of might have concerns. You need to **address these concerns and deflect any criticism.**

This candidate has done this by stating that she has dealt with her social group's lack of understanding. In one sentence she has cleverly shown she's able to deal with criticism of being 'interested in midwifery at an early age' **and** shown she's earned her friends' and family's support.

Try to list some of your most impressive hobbies: fishing and live music are good examples of having outside interests (fishing especially shows patience, practical skill, etc.). Additionally, mentioning that friends think you are a suitable candidate suggests this candidate is mature for her age.

"I have given thought to the long hours and shift work involved and feel I have the skills necessary to achieve a good work/life balance long term, based on the time I spent on the ward."

Mentioning you have thought through the shift work aspect of midwifery is good to mention, as this is a reason students often drop out, especially if they are expecting a normal university experience. The ultimate proof is offered here as the candidate has undertaken shift work on a ward. 'Work/life balance' is a buzz phrase in many professions at the moment and it is excellent to explore within your statement how you will achieve this.

"I understand midwifery is a career which many people want to join. I'd like to finish by saying that all I can bring you is a passion for the subject, motivation, a keen interest in the way midwifery care changes based on society and an appreciation of how much impact the professional relationship between midwife and women can have."

The candidate has offered a modest appraisal of what she can offer to the profession here. The 'all I can offer' will remind the admissions tutors of the candidate's acknowledgment that midwifery is challenging. The rest of the summary will remind them of the candidate's suitable skills and individual appeal. An enthusiasm for the profession with reference to the statement's opening paragraph about holistic partnership of care offers an easy to read, balanced ending.

Personal Statement Example 3: Excellent Technique From A 'Mature Student'

This final personal statement shows further excellent techniques which you can employ. In some ways the candidate has a more difficult statement to write as she has to sum up her complex life experience. Whether you're applying as a school leaver, or a mature candidate, these strategies can help you add a further edge to the effectiveness of your statement.

'You are braver than you believe, stronger than you seem, and smarter than you think.' That's a quote from A.A.Milne's 'Pooh's Grand Adventure' that I was reading to one of my children years ago, and it was at that moment the desire to be a midwife crystallised in my mind. It seemed a quote not only applicable to me, but to many mothers.

I became a mother as a teenager, and though bright, fell into some difficult circumstances. I am lucky to have a supportive family, and though I suffered from low academic confidence for years, when my children were old enough I worked full time in retail and simultaneously got my GCSEs. Then to my surprise I adored my 'Midwifery Access to Higher Education' course at college; my grades were more than adequate and I found studying with the prospect of being a midwife one day highly motivating. I was fascinated by the physiology module as it filled many gaps in my knowledge, and though challenging, I 'learnt how to learn'.

I am especially fascinated by waterbirth, and though my current Access Course does not cover the intricacies of care, I have done a lot of reading on the subject and found the amount of research staggering. I have read journal articles on the subject; finding the Cochrane library through my course has been illuminating. It's obvious there is more research needed on the subject, but overall, waterbirth seems to decrease intervention without adverse effects. Suggestions from French obstetrician Michel Odent that our evolutionary history of living in and out of water is an explanation of why waterbirth has such a massive impact on decreased intervention was exciting to read.

I worked in a clothes shop for many years while my children were growing up. This job contained many unsocial and long hours under time pressure, which has parallels with midwifery. I developed the ability to be personable and manage challenging behaviour from customers and staff, and progressed to be an area manager. I also came into contact with several vulnerable women in my workplace who I had to offer professional support to as manager. The ability to listen, take in incredibly complex and sad accounts of lives and act accordingly are life skills I value and feel are crucial tools for a midwife, even one in training.

I was lucky enough to shadow a community midwife for a week, which was enlightening. I can appreciate the different styles of care midwives must provide, from giving confidence and assurance to young mothers, to practical, language and medical help for refugees and immigrants, to the sensitive yet essential information which obese women need. I would have loved the opportunity to work on a labour ward, but I feel I understand the role of a midwife much more, not least in seeing how exhausting and frustrating it must be one day, yet rewarding and exciting on another. In the last year I have volunteered as an assistant in an Emergency Assessment Unit, which has given me insight into how NHS wards work. I was relieved to find I was up to the challenge of learning new skills like making beds, helping with bed baths and assisting patients with meals. The pace of NHS wards is fast; I felt my background in retail was adequate training for this.

I have a fantastic family life with both my parents and partner's parents involved. We enjoy sailing and walking. In my spare time I like to keep up with my friends by doing Belly Dancing (to my children's horror!). I am appreciative that my family and friends are so supportive about my desire to be a student midwife, and they help so I can study and work. I have thought hard about the impact on family life, and truly think we can manage well as a family unit.

I have good appreciation of how oversubscribed midwifery is thanks to my Access Course. However I hope my experience, fascination with the woman-centred approach of midwifery, sense of humour and determination will speak for me in my application.

Personal Statement Example 3: Analysis

In some ways this candidate has a harder job to do writing her statement than the candidate just out of school. Her professional life has been in retail, she has faced academic and life challenges and has not taken a traditional route to becoming a midwife. However the statement stands out, as it is crammed full of confidence. Her strong points are presented well and her weaker ones are turned into advantages.

" You are braver than you believe, stronger than you seem, and smarter than you think.' That's a quote from A.A.Milne's 'Pooh's Grand Adventure' that I was reading to one of my children years ago, and it was at that moment the desire to be a midwife

crystallised in my mind. It seemed a quote not only applicable to me, but to many mothers."

This opening paragraph quotes an unusual source and has a **story which draws attention.** From the beginning it is interesting, which is great news for a tired admissions tutor who has a pile of personal statements, many of which have the opening line 'From a young age I have wanted to be a midwife...'

(If you are thinking of using a quote in your statement, you should read the information in the Analysis of Personal Statement 1 before doing so, as there are some important points to consider.)

Life experience has prompted this candidate to take the first steps. This determination does her credit, and she understands part of a midwife's job is to **empower.**

"I became a mother as a teenager, and though bright, fell into some difficult circumstances."

Unfortunately some people, perhaps even prospective interviewers who should know better, will be quick to criticise teenage mothers. This candidate has cleverly presented this information with a positive aspect of her character: she is 'bright'.

"I am lucky to have a supportive family, and though I suffered from low academic confidence for years, as soon as my children were old enough I worked fulltime in retail and simultaneously got my GCSEs. Then to my

surprise I adored my 'Midwifery Access to Higher Education' course at college; my grades were more than adequate and I found studying with the prospect of perhaps being a midwife one day highly motivating."

Having a supportive family is, as discussed above, something interviewers look for, and is worth getting into your statement early, especially if you have family commitments. Describing 'low academic confidence' instead of saying you are 'not great at studying' or 'have had problems' is professionally put and crucially shows the candidate is reflective enough to know academic success depends on her self-belief and commitment. She then goes on to **show** rather than tell that she is able to do academic work around childcare as she was able to get her GCSEs. **This juggling of family, work and academic life also hints at excellent organisational skills.**

As discussed previously, it is important to show enthusiasm for academic work. Even if you class yourself as more of a practical person, there should be an area of academic midwifery that interests you enough to discuss it in your personal statement. (A note if you find academic work hard: many of the best midwives I have worked with have been people who find essays, research and so on hard. These midwives include some I'd love to have looking after me during labour! **It's OK to find things challenging, and everyone will find something on a midwifery course that is out of their comfort**

zone. Present the best you have to offer academically in a positive light and then concentrate on your other attributes if this is the case for you.)

It is obvious from this candidate's description of grades being 'more than adequate' that she is not top of the class. This is a positive way of describing average grades. It also indicates the candidate's motivation to accomplish even when challenged.

"I was fascinated by the physiology module as it filled many gaps in my knowledge, and though challenging, I 'learnt how to learn'."

Brilliant! A degree is a step up from an Access to HE or A-level course; you will not be 'spoon-fed' information but have to learn for yourself.

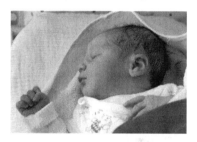

In some ways the difficulty this candidate has had will benefit her in a midwifery degree.

"I am especially fascinated by waterbirth, and though my current Access Course does not cover the intricacies of care, I have done a lot of reading on the subject and found the amount of research staggering. I have read journal articles on the subject; finding the Cochrane library through my course has been illuminating. It's obvious there is more research needed on the subject,

but overall waterbirth seems to decrease intervention without adverse effects."

Reading up on waterbirth is above and beyond the expected requirements for this candidate's course, and is impressive. The Cochrane library is a collection of high quality summaries and reviews of medical research; **the systematic reviews are free to view and the summaries only take a few minutes to read yet mentioning Cochrane is worth a lot in the eyes of an admissions tutor.** Crucially, this candidate has not only read the research but has been able to rationally criticise it, demonstrating above average understanding for a prospective student midwife.

The candidate has used a really handy tip that can be called upon when talking about most pieces of research - they have said more data is needed! This is an appropriate **criticism in the vast majority of research reports.** However, make sure you are able to talk in your interview about why more data is needed - as always, **don't write anything you are not happy to be quizzed about!**

"Suggestions from French obstetrician Michel Odent that our evolutionary history of living in and out of water is an explanation of why waterbirth has such a massive impact on decreased intervention was exciting to read."

This paragraph shows genuine excitement and a greater depth of reading. It is also an interesting theory in itself which is always useful - you want your admissions tutors to be captivated.

"I worked in a clothes shop for many years while my children were growing up. This job contained many unsocial and long hours, under time pressure, which has parallels with midwifery. I developed the ability to be personable and manage challenging behaviour from customers/staff, and progressed to be an area manager. I also came into contact with several vulnerable women in my workplace who I had to offer professional support to as manager. The ability to listen, take in incredibly complex and sad accounts of lives, and act accordingly are life skills I value and feel are crucial tools for a midwife, even one in training."

Mentioning how you will cope with unsocial and long hours is of benefit. This candidate presents **transferable skills** from her current job. Managing 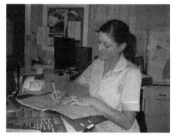 challenging behaviour from the public is a major skill in midwifery. The pastoral aspects of her job as a manager also have parallels with midwifery. She also demonstrates she is good at **listening**, which is an underrated yet brilliant skill for a student midwife to have.

"I was lucky enough to shadow a community midwife for a week, which was enlightening. I can appreciate the different styles of care midwives must provide, from confidence and assurance given to young mothers, to practical, language and medical help for refugees and immigrants, to the sensitive yet essential information obese women need. I would have loved the opportunity to work on a labour ward, but I feel I understand the role of a midwife much more; not least I can see how exhausting and frustrating it must be one day - yet rewarding and exciting on another."

This candidate has managed to get some directly applicable training and demonstrates she understands the role of a midwife well. She covers a range of complex situations with the age-old issue of midwifery support needed for refugees, to the more contemporary issue of obesity. She draws attention to the need for individualised care, which is an idea being examined in major research and guidelines currently. The last sentence in this paragraph shows that the candidate understands the challenges that come with being a midwife.

"In the last year I have volunteered as an assistant in an Emergency Assessment Unit, which has given me insight into how NHS wards work. I was relieved to find I was up to the challenge of learning new skills like making beds, helping with bed baths and assisting patients with meals. The pace of NHS wards is fast; I

felt my background in retail was adequate training for this.

The candidate over her statement has shown persistent commitment to her goal of training as a midwife; not only has she in her own time caught up on grades and done an Access to HE Course, she has shadowed a community midwife and volunteered on an NHS ward, all around family responsibilities. Skills picked up while volunteering are beneficial and the ability to learn on a 'fast paced' ward as a volunteer is also impressive.

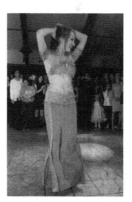

"I have a fantastic family life with both my parents and partner's parents involved. We enjoy sailing and walking. In my spare time I like to keep up with my friends by doing Belly Dancing (to my children's horror!). I am appreciative that family and friends are so supportive about my desire to be a student midwife, and they help so I can study and work. I have thought hard about the impact on family life and truly think we can manage well as a family unit."

A good social and family life is a very reassuring fact for the interviewers to hear. Outside interests also show a well-rounded applicant (no humour intended re the Belly Dancing). This candidate has also thought through her family commitments.

"I have good appreciation of how oversubscribed midwifery is thanks to my Access Course. However I hope my experience, fascination with the woman-centred approach of midwifery, sense of humour and determination speak for me in my application."

This last paragraph shows an understanding of the competition. This addresses the question that is often asked at interviews: 'Why should we give you a place over the other prospective students?' The candidate has summed up her major attributes to remind the admissions tutors what she has to offer and ends on a positive yet modest note.

With the tools in this chapter you will be able to put together a statement that showcases your abilities. You will need to draft and edit your personal statement a fair few times over a few weeks. Reading it after a few days' break might help you see it from the point of view of others (with fresh eyes).

As an aside, I advise you not to publish your personal statement online as it makes it easy for others to plagiarise. I have anecdotal evidence of a prospective student midwife who was accused of plagiarism as her personal statement had been copied by other candidates. It's not likely to be stolen, but it's probably not worth the risk.

Good luck and remember you can come and ask questions or see more material, including another personal statement example, and free videos, on MidwifeDiaries.com!

Chapter Three: Nervousness And How To Handle It

Introduction

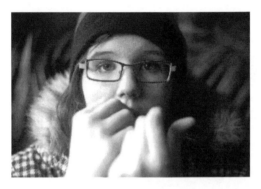

This chapter purposefully comes before the chapter on *"Panel Interview Technique"*. This is because when it comes to interviews:

"Midwives in the making know it - but they also have to show it!"

One of the most important ways you can prepare for your interview is by learning how to cope with your **emotional response**. It's really easy to do lots of preparation on midwifery, and despite this feel terrified walking into the interview room. We've all been there!

Most candidates (including me back in the day) will spend a minimal amount of time thinking about how they will cope emotionally. But if you're reading this book, **it's very likely that getting onto a midwifery course means a lot to you.**

If you are interviewing for a career that's important to you, you are likely to have adrenaline in your system. A misplaced 'fight or flight' reaction is likely, and can cause even the most prepared, suitable candidate to underperform! **The ability to handle this reaction is likely to be missing from your skillset at the moment.** It certainly was from mine when I was interviewing to become a student midwife.

The techniques in this chapter are based on the psychology evidence base and they really work - and work without making your answers appear staged or overconfident.

I should tell you here that I was very nervous at the start of my midwifery journey. Two of my own interviews went appallingly, I couldn't think and I shook and stuttered! But using these techniques I got excellent at midwifery interviews and now really enjoy interviews, even though my initial gut reaction to them hasn't changed.

Whether you are extremely nervous and know you need to get a handle on your interview skills, or you are an extrovert who's very happy being interviewed, the following techniques will help you come across as an excellent midwife in the making.

You'll also find out later in this chapter how my acronym '**DOPE**' can help you stay cool, calm and focussed in your interview.

Chronic Nervousness and Anxiety

(Before I address chronic nervousness, you should know that being afraid of interviewing to start with is fine - it can be incredibly compelling and make you perform extremely well.)

If you are severely affected by nerves and you get a dry mouth, sweaty palms and dizziness during interviews, you are likely to have an **introverted personality**. This is not a bad thing!

Many more people are introverts than you'd expect - roughly 50% of the population, according to Susan Cain, author of *'Quiet: The Power of Introverts in a World That Can't Stop Talking'*. A quote of hers that I love is: *'There's zero correlation between being the best talker and having the best ideas'* - you just need to work out your **style** in an interview situation.

If you fit into this category it may be you are a quiet, empathetic person with a lot to offer as a healthcare professional. Please don't give up just because interviews are not your thing - I've got you covered. Just follow the advice and give yourself lots of time.

Techniques and Using DOPE in Your Interview

Don't Fight With Your Emotions

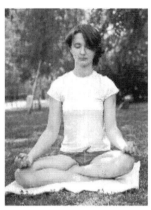

You're walking into your interview with good posture and grace. Your interview begins - and you are asked a question you are unprepared for!

You start to sweat, your scalp prickles and your mind goes blank. If you are like most of us, you dig deep, and try hard to think through the question. You struggle to keep your heart rate down and you tense, breathing fast.

But suppressing what you're experiencing **is not going to help.**

If you begin to have a 'fight or flight' reaction, try to identify exactly what it feels like. Take a few big breaths. Is there a buzzing in your tummy? Do you have tingles up and down your spine? Can you feel your heart beating?

If you don't fight with your emotions and merely try to feel exactly and precisely what's going on **whatever you are feeling will recede within 60 seconds or so.** All that energy will turn into a different emotion - excitement, interest, even calm.

This technique will allow your body to relax again. If you answer questions while truly experiencing what you're feeling, you will also come across as genuine and your answers will appear well thought out and heartfelt. Be comfortable in your own skin even if you're afraid. **Your interviewers will see you are a bit nervous - but they will want to cheer you on.**

If you continue trying to suppress your emotions, you are much more likely to waste energy and answer without thinking through properly, or even worse, come across as not genuine. This technique is also very useful for extroverts, to make you personable and to add more credibility to your answers!

This is a technique you need to practise, so I would suggest using your college or university 'mock interview' process to try it out. These are usually offered free, and you should have a couple of tries. You can also get friends and family to do mock interviews with you.

Neuro-Linguistic Programming

Many careers advisers suggest neuro-linguistic programming to help you feel confident and positive during intense situations like interviews. If you haven't come across neuro-linguistic programming before, it's an approach to making new behavioural patterns that can help achieve goals. This sounds intense, but all it really means is reprogramming your mind to think calmly about your interview process.

Some techniques from neuro-linguistic programming are not evidence based. There are plenty of things within this style of psychotherapy that I don't agree with - but some are truly excellent.

Visualisation is one of these. Visualisation is a technique that has been adopted by most elite athletes to help with their performance under pressure. You can use the technique too.

Spend around half an hour each day in the two weeks leading up to your interview imagining the whole process going smoothly. You can do this meditation style sitting with your eyes closed, before you go to bed at night, or while you're commuting. Whatever works for you is fine.

Vividly imagine what all your senses will experience on interview day; what you will hear (your excellent answers), what you will see (engaged and captivated interviewers), what you will smell (your lovely new smart clothes and a building that makes you comfortable), and feel (handing over all your correct paperwork).

It doesn't matter if you don't achieve all this on the day - the point is to make it all less scary. It's very likely this technique will help you get clear on how you want to appear in your interview, which will aid your whole preparation. It may even help you enjoy the process of being interviewed!

Power Posing

Sociologically, humans tend to prefer self-confident
(though not arrogant) people. Your interviewers will
be no different and this is a research-based and quick
way to increase your self-confidence. This will be
useful not only for the interview process but also
during your training as a student midwife.

When I first heard about 'power posing', my (very
British) cringe gland went into spasm. But despite the
slight connotations of bad life-coaching, this high
quality research comes from Harvard business school
and has a real physiological effect on stress and
nervousness.

The premise is that space-occupying, dominant poses
like those pictured, even if done for as little as 2
minutes, can have a positive impact on how you
interview. They are shown to reduce cortisol (a stress
hormone) and increase testosterone (a masculine
hormone).

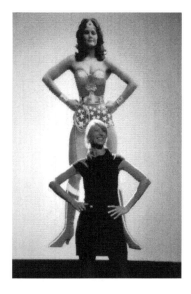

The effects of power posing are subtle. It will not make you appear arrogant - in the research interviewers could not identify candidates who had participated in power posing - but they did **rate candidates who have practised power posing as higher performing**. Not only that; power posing affects the way you feel to some extent, which will have a big impact on your ability to answer questions and think clearly. Feeling courageous is half the battle.

There is a useful free 'TED lecture' (the TED organisation offers excellent evidence-based lectures from experts) on the subject at:

www.ted.com/talks/amy_cuddy_your_body_languag e_shapes_who_you_are

So in those nerve wracking few minutes while you are
waiting to be called into the interview room, why not
pop to the toilet and do some power posing!

Equality Philosophy

As I've got older and developed as a practitioner, I
have developed a logic-based belief which is useful
when dealing with managers, doctors, or any other
people that might be understood to be more
authoritative than me. I have found this incredibly
beneficial in interviews and work situations.

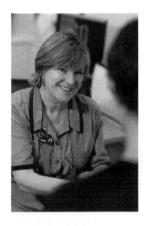

It is simply this: **truly believe
you are equal to your
interviewers**. Do not aim to
get their approval - just do the
best job you can do. You are
applying to be a student
midwife with good intentions
of being in a caring profession.
You're not arrogant for
interviewing. You have not
chosen your upbringing, life
experience, and other qualities, meaning you have
**every right to converse on a level with your
interviewer.**

You had little choice in who you are today, but you
might develop tomorrow into an excellent midwife.
**You might even be more successful or
knowledgeable than them one day!** Be polite, but

know you are their equal and might have something
to add to their knowledge already.

For me and others this opens possibilities that do not
exist when feeling a bit inferior. It's hard to answer
questions if you are constantly focused on
interviewers knowing the topic better than you do.

I find having this **philosophy of equality** to be the
icing on the cake when it comes to coping with
nervousness or fear. Combined with the other coping
strategies, you can improve your performance no end.

Use DOPE:

To help you remember all your steps when you are in
an interview situation, calm down and use the **DOPE**
acronym:

D - Don't fight with your emotions

O - Use your neurO-linguistic programming

P - Power Posing

E - Equality Philosophy

All of these techniques are helpful, but I hope you
manage to apply the 'Don't Fight With Your
Emotions' point most of all, as it's the queen of all
tips to get your nervousness under control. After that
you can bolster your confidence and performance
with the other techniques.

Chapter Four: Panel Interview Technique

How To Dress And How To Show Your Composure On Interview Day

Panel Interview Technique is one of the essential skillsets you need to secure a place as a student midwife.

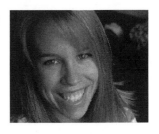

Whether you're already comfortable with interviews and just need to bring your experience together in a midwifery context, or are just starting to learn interview technique and don't know where to begin, this information will help you show you are an excellent candidate.

When I was applying to be a midwife, I went to almost everyone I knew about my impending interviews to get over my nerves and get some help. I was talking to a friend of mine who happens to have (high functioning) autism. His autism seems to allow him to cut to the truth of matters sometimes. He said *'All you have to do is go in and show them you're not a mad axe murderer. You have a bit of experience, you can cope with the academic stuff and you really care about women. What more could they want? It's not rocket science.'*

This thought really helped me - most of us overcomplicate things.

This chapter is designed to teach you interview techniques without seeming overconfident, overexcited, or overwrought - it's about drawing out skills you have already, adding extra midwifery knowledge, and learning how to demonstrate your suitability to your interviewers.

Dress And Composure

Most interviews for professionals call for a smart appearance and midwifery is no different. Casual office wear is very appropriate. Make sure you are comfortable in your outfit. **Did you know research suggests interviewers make up their mind about candidates within the first 30 seconds?** The way you dress will obviously have an impact on their decision.

For women: Black, brown or grey trousers, an ironed shirt or top, not low cut. Sensible shoes - black or brown, small/no heel. I personally would opt for trousers as you may have to do an active group task.

For men: Black or brown trousers, an ironed shirt, tidy hair tied back or cut short. Black or brown smart work shoes.

Have clean, short nails and good personal hygiene. Wearing a watch can hint you care about timekeeping.

Your average UK midwife will wear a uniform or scrubs, with their hair short or tied back. They will avoid any jewellery other than a small pair of stud earrings, and perhaps a wedding ring. This is due to infection control. They will often not wear heavy makeup as it's impractical when working in hot or wet environments (for instance attending waterbirth - no, you are not expected to get in the pool! But it's often a bit steamy and you can get splashed).

I would imitate this as much as is practical. You are trying to persuade your interviewer you would fit in as a midwife. Even if it only registers with them subconsciously that you look a bit like their colleagues or students already training, you have gained an advantage.

Posture: Stand upright and walk confidently in front of your interviewers. Even if you're secretly shaking in your shoes, they won't be able to tell if you keep a relaxed posture. Sean Connery got the part of James Bond as the director saw him walking down the street 'moving like a panther', and this isn't so far off what you should aim for (though it's not in your best interests to drop on all fours and growl). Remember to smile as well, as it shows you're confident.

Language: Aim for simple language with straightforward meaning. Don't waffle - if you can help it. **If you are nervous, slow down and aim for clarity, don't speed up.**

For instance in answer to 'why do you want to be a midwife?' answering with a long winded story about your experience of family being looked after by midwives has a less obvious meaning than: 'I am interested in supporting women through normal, healthy life events. It motivates me more than any other aspect of healthcare'.

Most of us try and use big words when we are interviewing to make us seem intelligent. But research (published in *Psychology Today* by Daniel Oppenheimer) suggests using simple rather than complex language actually makes us appear cleverer. Instead of saying 'I am deeply interested in midwifery and spend time perusing textbooks and journals to better my knowledge', just say 'I love reading about midwifery. Textbooks, blogs, journals, NICE guidelines - it's all fascinating to me'.

Eye contact: Give your interviewers eye contact from time to time. Space this between your interviewers to show you are comfortable but don't outstare them. It's worth saying again: **remember to smile!**

Prepare: Being prepared will aid your confidence and persuade your interviewers you are an excellent candidate. Read the sample questions and answers in Chapter Seven: *"Practice Questions And Answers"*. Have a friend interview you and record yourself on camera to see what can be improved. Highlight bits of this chapter which you find useful and read them through a few times. It's worth knowing you will not be expected to provide in depth clinical answers as you have not had training - having basic knowledge and common sense will be enough.

Practicalities: Make sure you have the required paperwork listed on the information sheet the university will give you. This usually means certificates, passport photos and perhaps other documents. Having all the right bits and pieces is an easy way to impress them within **that crucial first 30 seconds.**

Essential Knowledge

Being a midwife comes with many legal and personal responsibilities, which means even as an applicant you should know the main organisations that govern, advise 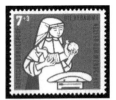 and work for midwives. There are three organisations that you should know about. Spending ten minutes or so on the website (or Wikipedia page!) of each of these would give you the information you need to know. In summary:

The Nursing and Midwifery Council (NMC): www.nmc-uk.org The NMC protects the public. It publishes codes for nurses and midwives that must be adhered to, it keeps a register of midwives, addresses complaints, and has the power to remove practitioners from its registers. Basically, it regulates midwives.

The Royal College of Midwives (RCM): www.rcm.org.uk This is the trade union for midwives (the only UK trade union for midwives). It is optional to join the union (for a fee), and it offers legal and educational support and campaigns for various good 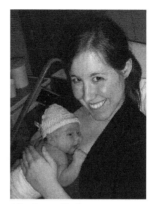 things for maternity care and midwives. It has a fascinating history you might like to look at.

The National Institute for Health and Care Excellence (NICE): www.nice.org.uk This is a branch of the Department of Health but exercises a lot of independent power. It lays down excellent guidelines for health care, taking into account funds available within the NHS and all available evidence and research.

The 5 Questions You Should Prepare For

Work smart not hard. It can be tempting to try and prepare for every eventuality, but it's unlikely you will have time, and besides, every candidate will feel underprepared in some way walking into the interview. Try to get a broad overview of what could be asked and what attitude you need to have. Be able to have a shot at any question based on common sense, your own knowledge and what you have specifically revised.

Remember, if you are nervous, slow down, don't speed up. The odds are you already know the answer or at least a good response!

Have answers planned for at least the questions below. I have included example answers.

1. *What is the role of a midwife?*

The role of a midwife, in summary, is to be highly skilled in caring for women and their babies throughout the antenatal, intrapartum and postnatal period (and in some cases the women in the prenatal period). They focus on normality, and midwifery care appears to decrease maternal and infant mortality and morbidity as opposed to obstetric care alone. As healthcare professionals who independently look after normally progressing pregnancies, midwives must command a broad range of knowledge and be able to refer to the medical team in case of any deviations from normal and to offer first line treatment in emergency situations. They also have a key role in breastfeeding and infant health. Some midwives specialise in areas like teenage pregnancy, diabetes, bereavement and so on. Some midwives focus on normality in birth centres and in the community.

2. *Why do you want to be a midwife?*

That's a huge question. I want to be a midwife because pregnancy, birth and the postnatal period fascinate me. I think midwives are onto something in the way they offer holistic care for women, from social and emotional help all the way to the analysis of fetal heart rates. I think what they offer amounts to true health care, and helping women have their babies in an empowering way, I think, can affect whole societies. I am passionate, tough and very organised and I think my personality is suited towards ongoing challenges. I'm happiest when challenged.

3. *How will you cope with the pressure of training and being a midwife?*

Well, as I said, I'm happiest when challenged. That's not to say I don't take my work/life balance seriously. Anyone can get burnt out. I would try to put everything into perspective and see it as all adding up to giving good care for women. The thought of the responsibility is overwhelming and I'm not sure anyone can truly understand what that's like until they are doing it, but I would rather be doing this than applying myself to a business or something relatively inconsequential.

I also have a very supportive family and a good friendship group. We like rock climbing, and I'd try and get that in as much as possible for stress relief. The nice thing about rock climbers is there tends to be someone at the climbing wall very early in the morning and very late at night as they try and fit it around work, so there would always be someone to talk to and climb with, even around shifts.

4. *What are the key bodies that govern and advise midwives in the UK?*

The Nursing and Midwifery Council is the organisation that governs midwives. They publish 'codes' which are strict rules and guidelines that must be adhered to, covering everything from practice to personal conduct. They also have the power to take people off the register.

NICE, the National Institute for Health Care and Excellence examines research and comes up with best practice guidelines for the UK.

The Royal College of Midwives is the Midwifery Trade Union, which helps campaign for better care for women and a better working environment for midwives. They launched a 'Campaign for Normal Birth' in 2005 to address these issues, as they believe medicalisation is detracting from women's care. They have lots of resources on their website to promote normal birth, and lobby for more midwives in the UK as well as better funding.

In terms of other key bodies there's the Cochrane library which offers systematic reviews of evidence and the Royal College of Obstetricians which offer clinical guidelines which sometimes cover more medicalised subjects in greater depth.

5. *What will your weaknesses and strengths be in training as a midwife?*

I am passionate about giving good care to women. This is an advantage as it increases my motivation. But it's also a weakness, as I understand it is very difficult to give perfect care when there are such pressures on the service. I would try very hard to put everything in perspective and see care in terms of managing the women in my care as a whole. Having said that, I know I would also try and improve individual client experiences on a case by case basis, just by using a combination of perspective and trying to intelligently use the resources I had available, I suppose!

My strengths in general are my compassionate nature even under time pressure, my attention to detail, and my motivation to be an excellent practitioner.

Research Your University

If you can, tailor your preparation to the specific university you are applying to. Know facts and a few stats and be able to discuss the topic of the moment in the local maternity unit. This can be an easy way to give yourself an edge over the competition. You can do this by:

• Going to a university open day and asking student midwives or prospective interviewers what successes and contentious issues the trust currently enjoys and faces. For instance, is there a particular area of research going on? Is the maternity unit suited to rural/urban services, dealing with a record number of births in a year, or does it have a specialist philosophy like available one-on-one midwifery care?

• Have a look at the midwifery section of hospital websites to see what you can find. Similarly, get onto studentmidwivessanctuary.com, search for your prospective hospital or university and see what comes up. Your interviewers will be impressed if you can say something like '(Birmingham) has an excellent reputation for its new birth pools. I am very interested in waterbirth and can't wait to find out more.'

• Ring the university in question and ask specifically who is on the panel. You may be able to find out their special interest subject and tailor your interview accordingly. Do they think bladder care is the most important thing about midwifery? Have they written a paper on teenage pregnancy you can nonchalantly refer to? Do they like or loathe homebirth? This is powerful information for you. You might be refused, but it is unlikely to lessen your chances of getting a place. Even if the interviewer in question finds out you have been trying to work out who they are, this can only be in your favour as it shows enthusiasm and initiative.

• Try to find a midwife or student midwife from your target university and talk to her - perhaps you could take her out for coffee and try and get as much useful advice as you can!

Use Of Humour

Unlike in your personal statement, when you are face to face with interviewers, humour can be extremely useful. Meeting anyone for the first time is usually socially demanding. Humour is often used in these situations to 'melt the ice', and a formal interview 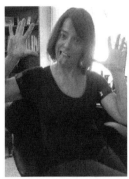 setting is no different! It can also help you to present yourself as approachable and intelligent and can help you to show your personality (which if your interviewers have already seen 250 people that week can be a real asset).

If it doesn't feel right to make a joke then don't - you will usually be able to read a lot from your interviewers about the appropriateness. If you don't joke around naturally then you might not feel comfortable cracking a joke, and that's fine too.

Things to avoid:

• Sarcasm - not necessarily the lowest form of wit, but be careful. The interviewers don't know you, and could think you are being serious! This may cause offence (especially if your interviewer happens to be from a culture which doesn't include a lot of irony or sarcasm).

• Swearing - not appropriate in an interview situation. Swearing while working as a midwife is not appropriate, so it's best to steer clear.

• Anything that could cause offence to a minority group by referring to ethnicity, sexuality, race, class, etc.

• Constant jokes: one or two moments of humour can be brilliant, but don't make every other sentence amusing. The interviewers need to see you being serious as well or they won't be able to understand your personality and suitability.

'Is There Anything You Want To Ask?' - How To Question Your Interviewer

Your interviewers will usually round off by asking if there is anything you want to ask. You can take this opportunity to ask some interesting questions about the university, the course, or midwifery in general. Use this time to find out what you want to know - but also to show you are an engaged, interesting and motivated candidate. Example questions include:

• How does the university approach normality in pregnancy and childbirth?

• What postgraduate options do you offer?

• How do you think the midwifery staffing deficit will resolve?

• Do students do community placements?

• How do you support students on delivery suite?

If you don't have any questions or the ones you had have been answered during the interview then say something like; 'I had lots when I walked through the door but you've already answered them. Thank you.'

Further content:

You might find the free posts and content at midwifediaries.com/category/resources-for-prospective-student-midwives/prospective-student-midwives/ useful for your interview. I keep the information up to date with current trends in interviewing.

The Evening Before And Day Of Your Interview

An excellent guide from the University of Cumbria website, that summarises everything interviewers look for, can be found here reproduced on MidwifeDiaries.com: midwifediaries.com/midwifery-interview-specification/

It's a specification mark scheme used to assess candidates and it might bring together your thoughts on how to perform in your interview. You may want to look at this the night before your interview.

If you are interviewing in your own town, have a dry run and work out where the university building is. If not, plan your journey well. If the interview is early in the morning and a few hours' drive away, consider staying in town overnight, which will also give you the opportunity to see if you like the area.

I would suggest getting some good cardiovascular exercise the day before your interview. I would also suggest a good night's sleep and sensible meals without too much caffeine or sugar for dinner and breakfast (staying in town before your interview might also be a good idea if you have a busy home life...not everyone will have this luxury but if you can manage it, you may benefit from being relaxed the night before.)

There's no point in getting too het up at this point - you've done your preparation, you know your reasons for wanting to join in and be useful as a midwife, the answers will come! If you're feeling nervous, move back to the previous chapter for lots of easy to implement help.

You can also always come and get some support on **'The Secret Community For Midwives in the Making'**, which you can join via Facebook.

Try not to stress after your interview. It's really hard to judge how things went - you can over-analyse for days. There can be all kind of reasons you don't hear back from your university quickly, and they might not have anything to do with you.

I know it's really hard, and I remember being on tenterhooks for weeks. But if you can take philosophical advice from *The Beatles* once you've finished your interview - '*Let it be*'.

Chapter Five: Above And Beyond

By reading the previous chapters you should have enough information to present yourself as an attractive candidate for your interviewers. There are, however, a few other techniques you can use to help the interviewers discriminate further in your favour.

Many of these techniques will work for people regardless of their personalities and attributes. However, you must feel comfortable with them, and they have to be sincere. Interviewers, just like anyone, will be able to spot continuous insincerity.

Used correctly, they can be very effective in showcasing the qualities that interviewers look for.

What Else Interviewers Look For

What exactly are you trying to achieve? You are trying to make your interviewers distinguish between you and the rest of the pack. You want to demonstrate that you are a very good choice.

Let's assess how your interviewers will be thinking:

Imagine yourself in their shoes. You are a busy midwife, have children, work part time, you lecture part time and you have many small projects ticking along. You might be doing a PhD or research. Sometimes your career brings you a sense of gratitude and joy. Other days you despair at the huge task in front of you and the midwifery staffing deficit whilst the birth rate in the UK is rising.

You are interviewing candidates. You have a personal statement, a 20-30 minute interview and perhaps a day of group interviews or other tests to help you decide who the midwives of the future are. **What are you looking for?**

The candidate will need to remain **passionate** even on longs days of academic study/essay writing. She or he will need to continue **empowering women** and eventually **lead other healthcare professionals**, even on days when she or he feels like everything has gone wrong. She or he will have to cope with an incredible amount of stress, hard work and responsibility. They will also be harshly criticised at some point in their training and career.

To summarise, the candidate must be:

• Academically able and organised

• Resistant to burnout

• Able to take constructive criticism while being resilient to unconstructive criticism

• Have sustainable passion, even when tired

To be viewed as exceptional, the candidate must convince you they have these capabilities. And they must do it clearly and succinctly as you have very limited time to think about each individual.

So you, as a candidate, do not have a particularly easy task, but it can be achieved and this chapter will help you!

Your Specialist Interest Subject

My first piece of advice is to choose a **specialist interest subject** within midwifery that fascinates you. This will help showcase your **academic ability** and to some extent your **resistance to burnout.**

Your specialist interest subject, as discussed before in this book, should be something you find fascinating.

Some ideas include:

• The impact of poverty on midwifery outcomes

• Teenage pregnancy

• Ethnic minorities and language barriers

• Obesity

• Waterbirth

• Mental Illness

You can use your specialist interest subject as a **springboard into midwifery literature and culture;**

reading around a subject like this will enable a **depth of understanding** that most other candidates will not be able to achieve. It should give you a flavour of the major themes and contentious issues that exist in midwifery.

For instance, the last example personal statement in Chapter Two featured a candidate who was very interested in waterbirth. She demonstrated her ability to read research, comment on contemporary theories, and showed how this was related to midwifery practice. It showcased her outstanding **academic ability** with a depth of understanding that is hard to achieve (unless you have focussed in on one particular area).

Her specialist interest subject also helped her prove her **resistance to burnout.** Her excitement about the topic was evident in her writing. It suggests she would enjoy knowing more about the subject - her passion for midwifery would be well placed and well used in a clinical placement.

Your specialist interest subject can also be used to suggest that you have thoughts about your **long term career prospects**. If you are interested in a specialist role, for instance diabetes educator, specialist teenage pregnancy midwife, child protection midwife, and so on, this can be a real encouragement as it suggests you **won't leave the profession after a few short years.**

To show consistency you could mention your specialist interest subject in your personal statement, in your personal interview, in your portfolio (more to come on this later), or anywhere else it feels applicable.

It is worth mentioning here that you should not shoehorn your subject into every situation, as it might come across as obsessional if you don't answer other interview questions. You want to talk about your specialist interest, but don't neglect any other area in favour of it. You need to be a well-rounded candidate; **your specialist interest subject is the icing on the cake.**

You should dedicate at least several hours to looking at your specialist interest subject in detail. You will almost **definitely be asked about it if it featured in your personal statement.** Write down what you learn, especially interesting points and insightful statistics. You may be presented with an opportunity to quote them in your interview which would be extremely impressive.

Some Resources For Learning About Your Specialist Interest Subject Include...

• A good old Google search, but don't underestimate the usefulness of Google Scholar either. See the 'Computer and Research Tricks' section in Chapter One, page 18, for more info about this.

• MidwifeDiaries.com has interesting articles and resources, and I try to keep it well stocked with up to date information.

• YouTube videos both of professional resources and homemade material (there are all kinds of births documented online and lots of lectures from various midwives and obstetricians).

• A search on the BBC website for news articles on your topic.

• NICE guidelines; as outlined earlier, NICE compiles evidence and presents guidelines for healthcare professionals. You can find them via the NICE wesbsite: www.nice.org.uk

• Statements and guidance from the Royal College of Midwives and Royal College of Obstetricians and Gynaecologists – all to be found on their respective websites.

• Cochrane reports, to be found at: www.thecochranelibrary.com

As explained in previous chapters, Cochrane offers some of the most up to date and comprehensive care evidence in the world, and is free. Cochrane evidence comes from systematic reviews, usually of high quality randomised controlled trials. This type of assessment of evidence is the most reliable sort available within research.

The library was named after Archie Cochrane, a Scottish Doctor who was interested in clear evidence behind treatment. 'Cochrane' is pronounced numerous ways but 'Coc-rin' seems to be the most widely accepted variant.

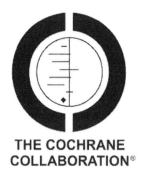

THE COCHRANE COLLABORATION®

The Cochrane Collaboration logo shown above is interesting and has a midwifery slant: it shows a **forest plot** of data which went on to inform many obstetricians about the effectiveness of **giving steroids to Mums in premature labour.** Before this, though the data was available, most obstetricians didn't know quite how effective it was. It has now become standard practice. The treatment increases the **likelihood of premature babies surviving by 30-50% as it develops their lungs,** and application of this fact through Cochrane has without doubt saved many babies' lives. Whip *that* piece of information out nonchalantly at your interviewers if you can!

• Studentmidwivessanctuary.com, the evidencebasedbirth.com and midwiferyonline.co.uk all offer forum searches which are very helpful.

• CEMACE stand for the 'Centre for Maternal and Child Enquiries'. It is a government organisation that looks into the reasons mothers and babies die every year. They issue a bi-annual report, and it's a key text for making maternity care better.

Confusingly they used to be called CEMACH (Confidential Enquiry into Maternal Deaths in the UK). The reports makes harrowing reading – but often highlight areas of care that need to be improved, making it an important source of information for you to understand your specialist interest subject. I can't give you an address as CEMACE don't have one specifically for their reports, instead they are usually, but not always, distributed via 'www.rcog.org.uk'. Failing that you will be able to find them with a simple Google search.

• Borrow from the library/buy a small, up to date book on your specialist interest subject and either read or skim read it. This will give you good insight and it will also be impressive to mention you have read it during your interview.

• Try to talk to a midwife, or a woman effected by the subject. The National Childbirth Trust might be able to help with this but you can always drop by MidwifeDiaries.com, or 'The Secret Community for Midwives in the Making' on Facebook and ask a specific question too. Alternatively you could find someone in your social circle to talk to.

• With this information, put together a few pages of your thoughts. This can include interesting statistics and research evidence, quotes, a small paragraph on your reflections, and notes on any interviews you have conducted. Present this professionally and with some useful pictures and put it into a folder.

Showing Your Resilience

It's difficult to show your ability to take constructive criticism in an interview situation. You may be feeling uncomfortable, meaning you're not really in the mood to talk to your interviewers about your resilience! However being able to process criticism during clinical practice, as well as being able to identify unfounded criticism are key tools for training successfully, and ones that are underestimated by most candidates.

Having prepared a story on your ability to deal with criticism, you may be able to identify something from your time doing work experience for midwifery, or in a previous job. For instance, a good story showcasing ability to deal with constructive criticism might be:

'It's important when you're working in a big department shop to take constructive criticism well and quickly. For instance when I was new to my shop, I signed for and took an order of some equipment. I didn't know the equipment was not allowed to be used for insurance reasons until all staff had been trained, and the equipment in question was being distributed all around the shop at once.

The colleague who criticised me did so quite sharply, and it would have been easy to feel embarrassed.

However logically, I couldn't have known what I didn't know! So I just rounded up all the equipment with some help from other colleagues, which wasn't really an easy task as I didn't know all the areas!

My colleague continued to give me a dressing down after the situation had resolved. However I felt I had learnt a lot about the way the shop ran and the procedures for accepting deliveries, and there was not much left to learn from the experience. In the end I had to thank her for letting me know the correct procedure, but tell her that ongoing criticism wasn't helping me get any better at my job....I know these situations happen in all walks of life but I suspect when training in a practical job like midwifery with so much responsibility these situations would crop up frequently. I'd like to think I can handle constructive criticism and benefit from it, and that I have the skills to handle less constructive criticism too!'

This story could fit into answering an interview questions such as:

• How would you deal with a disagreement with a colleague?

• What would be some of the most stressful parts of the course?

• Describe a time you have learnt from a mistake.

• What skills have you got that are transferable from other jobs?

• What do you think would be the hardest part of this job?

Of course, you need to give a well-rounded answer, so add your statement about criticism after you have addressed the question in any other way you think is necessary.

Your Portfolio

The last technique I suggest is to put together a small portfolio. A portfolio is a good medium to demonstrate your sustainable passion and determination.

All student midwives and qualified midwives keep portfolios, so it should help get you on the same wavelength as your interviewers. Some universities ask for a portfolio from all applicants but most do not. Merely having put it together should give you an edge when applying to the majority of universities. It should feature your passion and ongoing development as a prospective midwife.

An applicant's portfolio shouldn't be huge: Between 5 and 15 pages of notes and other bits and pieces is fine. Get a professional looking folder and make sure the presentation is neat.

I'm not suggesting you make a huge effort (the word 'portfolio' makes my own motivation sink to my shoes!), but make it exciting and about your passion for midwifery and by all means include plenty of pictures.

It should include:

• A few notes on your work experience and how it relates to midwifery

• A few lines on why you want to be a midwife

• A collection of materials on your chosen **specialist interest subject**

You can also put in all kinds of certificates that have transferable skills, as well as favourite articles, essays you might have written for courses that have a midwifery slant, anything you can think of that is appropriate! Be creative and let the portfolio be guided by what fascinates you.

There may be an opportunity to show your portfolio (off) in your interview, but the act of writing it should improve your chances significantly because it will get you thinking in the right way. You could also make a copy of it to take with you. Leave it at the end of your interview, telling your interviewers that it could address any other questions they might have.

To conclude:

If a midwife in the making came to an interview well dressed, was polite, answered most key questions in the interview well, had the right academic credentials, and was personable, they would be an attractive candidate to the interviewers.

However, if she or he showed academic ability for midwifery with a **specialist interest subject**, was able to keep a **clear head**, could obviously **handle** criticism and showed **sustainable passion for midwifery** and **drive** above other candidates demonstrated with a portfolio, she or he would be much more likely viewed as an **exceptional candidate.**

Chapter Six: Additional Selection Activities

This chapter will address the **other types of interview** that sometimes feature as part of the selection process. These differ depending on the 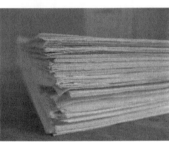 university, but there are some tricks you can learn to be able to approach any of these tests well, and some specifics for maths/literacy tests you should know about. It's important that you get a handle on these tests for a very good reason - I'll go into why this is at the end of this chapter.

Whether you're just starting to learn how to handle interviews and the thought of yet more activities to prepare for concerns you because you don't know how to begin, or you've been around the block in terms of interviewing but still aren't quite comfortable with these additional skills, this chapter will give you the inside information you need to do brilliantly.

It's easy to worry about preparing for these activities, especially as there are not many resources out there to help - but don't worry, this chapter and the next will set you up for success - and the main secret is **they are not hard if you do a bit of revision.**

Group Interviews

Group interview sessions usually last between 10-30 minutes. These activities are used to see how you behave around other people. You will likely be assessed for your **communication, leadership, negotiation** and **teamwork** skills.

Basics

• You will probably be asked to introduce yourself to the group, and give a little of your history. Choose a few key facts about yourself that show **leadership, responsibility,** or other transferable skills. Extra-curricular activities like orienteering, rock climbing, volunteer work and so on would be very good to mention! You can positively frame activities in your life, for instance: stating you love going out with your friends to live music gigs is much better than revealing you like to go out drinking lots of vodka with your mates, despite them being remarkably similar things - you get the idea!

• Your **body language** is important as what you say will be among many other voices. Power posing, as discussed on page 77, may be very useful before your group interview. Try to project a calm, confident posture, so don't sit with your arms crossed. If you are able to, and if it seems appropriate, lean forwards slightly. Make eye contact with other candidates, and exchange smiles.

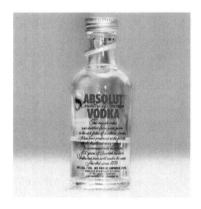

• **Do not dominate the conversation;** this is a common mistake in group interviews. However, if no-one seems able to direct the group, especially if you are asked to complete a task, gently delegate tasks or direct the conversation, using polite language (please and thank you).

• Make sure you practice **active listening skills** - these skills are so important. Answer topics brought up by group members.

• If you feel there is a valid point to be made which is **mildly controversial**, it could work in your favour to bring it up, as it shows individuality. For instance, you could say: 'Every woman has a right to her informed choice even if the decision goes against medical recommendations'

• Be the **mediator** if a controversy in the discussion continues.

• Bring up a new area for discussion if possible and it feels applicable.

• Make sure you **contribute to the discussion.**

• It would be beneficial to remember something another candidate said earlier in the day and bring it into the 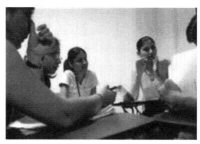 discussion to show you are socially aware. Show your genuine interest in other candidates.

• Remember - you are just as interesting and your views are just as valid as anyone else's!

If you come across as well rounded and proactive, and don't demonstrate any undesirable characteristics (for example, racism, homophobia, or a simple lack of ability to talk to others!) you are highly likely to pass your group interview with flying colours.

The secret to group interviews is: as long as you are not silent or really pushy, or say 'I think I'd only do the first year of training to get to deliver a baby' or something equally silly, you won't be able to do much wrong!

Group Interview questions may be on surprisingly random topics.

The following are real examples from group interviews:

• Your plane has crashed on a desert island. You have various supplies, a bit of drinking water and some equipment. How would you work together as a group to ensure your survival before being rescued?

• Read this information on global warming. Can you use these pens and paper to make a poster, and as a group present the information to the admissions tutors?

• Have a look at these photos which document a journey. Can you, as a group, order them in terms of how the story progresses?

• You have all been briefed to bring two photos showing you doing something in your life which has good transferrable skills to midwifery. Please exchange and discuss these photos and the qualities you think are important in midwives.

Midwifery specific group interview questions can be on anything - your answers to the these type of questions will be taken into account, but are not as important as how you are reacting in a group setting. More in depth questions will be left to your one on one interview.

Group interviews are usually supervised by a few interviewers, and perhaps a 'service user', i.e. a mother who has recently used maternity care services. Sometimes there might be midwives listening and assessing who are not involved with the rest of the interview process.

Overall, if you've prepared for your panel interview well, you will have more than enough info to get you through your group interview!

Presentations

Occasionally universities will ask you to put together a presentation of 5-10 minutes length to either present to the group of prospective candidates and interviewers, or just a panel of interviewers. You will usually be given at least a few weeks to prepare and they might ask you to use PowerPoint.

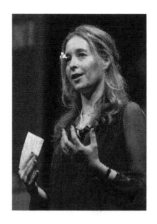

You will be able to find tutorials on how to use PowerPoint on YouTube, or on the Microsoft website.

The following are real examples of presentation topics set for candidates:

• How will you start to support childbearing women when you become a student midwife?

• What qualities do you think are important for midwives to have?

• What is the role of a midwife?

Your most important tactic for a good presentation is to give yourself **plenty of time to prepare** and **know how you will cope emotionally.** You can use the information on page 100 to research for answers to your set presentation, and try using the DOPE acronym from Chapter Three to help you give a calm and confident performance.

Basics:

• Make yourself flashcards; try not to have a script as you often just end up reading it out without engaging with the content.

• Do your presentation in front of family, friends and others a few times.

• Make sure your content works and be prepared to give your presentation without PowerPoint if it all goes wrong and your USB stick doesn't work - have PowerPoint there to add information and pictures, not to lead your presentation.

• Smile and have confidence.

• Be prepared for one or two questions on your presentation - have a few answers planned to possible questions, and be prepared to think on your feet for others. There's nothing wrong with saying **'I'd need to do a bit more research to answer that question to my satisfaction', as long as you have a go at a plausible answer.**

• Don't worry about having massively in depth midwifery knowledge or being right about everything - you have not trained as a midwife, and your interviewers will be looking for **potential** not **perfection.**

In interview presentations, once again my best advice is:

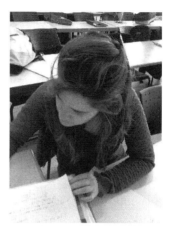

"Midwives in the making know it - but they also have to show it!"

With some confidence, some eye contact with members of your audience, a well-planned presentation, and some facts and insights at your fingertips, there's no reason why you shouldn't dazzle your interviewers.

Numeracy and Literacy Tests:

If you find maths or literacy challenging, you may be encouraged to know I've worked with loads of midwives who have dyscalculia (a learning disorder which involves difficulty working with numbers) or dyslexia (a similar disorder which affects language comprehension and use), and are excellent practitioners. Just because you start off with a disadvantage doesn't mean you can't master exactly what you need to!

Just remember: **there will be something challenging for everyone on a midwifery course as there are such diverse skills involved.**

You can speak to the university before your exam if you have a diagnosed condition which will affect your performance. They may be able to give you extra time or aid you in another way.

However, if you don't have a diagnosis it may be difficult for them to help you - think about trying to get formally diagnosed before your interview, or come up with your own coping strategy, for instance revising under time pressure or spending a few sessions with an English or Maths tutor.

The standards of maths and literacy tests are set by the Nursing and Midwifery Council (the governing body for midwives). You **only** have to prove you are safe to document notes and understand them, and handle and dispense drugs; you do not need to be a great writer or brilliant mathematician!

Numeracy Tests

These tend to be done without a calculator, though you may have to prove you can use one as well. They are basic and with a little preparation, there is no reason why you shouldn't pass easily.

If you revise the following you will be in a strong position:

• Digital and analogue time

• Decimals, ratios, percentages, fractions, and converting between them

• Conversion between litres and millilitres, kilograms, grams and milligrams

• Addition, subtraction, division, multiplication

• Basic statistics: mean, median, and mode

If you revise the following, you will be in an even stronger position:

• BODMAS

• Finding the square root of whole numbers

• Long addition

• Long subtraction

• Long multiplication

• Long division

The BBC Bitesize revision website offers an excellent guide to these calculations and includes questions and answers. It can be found at www.bbc.co.uk/schools/gcsebitesize/maths/

The BBC Skillswise website is also very useful and can be found at www.bbc.co.uk/skillswise/maths

Leeds University offers good free instruction on their website at library.leeds.ac.uk/tutorials/maths-quizzes/pages/nurses/

Sample numeracy tests with answers can be found in Chapter Seven. Perhaps time yourself doing the first test, work out which areas you find difficult before trying the second. The numeracy tests in Chapter Seven are representative of the hardest examples -

sorry about that, but some universities will set questions like this, so it is important to prepare for this level of difficulty!

A Google search for your particular university may well show you a sample test of the type that you'll have to take on the day, which can be really helpful.

Literacy Tests

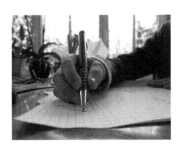

Literacy tests also test pretty basic skills. They come in a few different types depending on the university.

• The first type is a small essay to be written in 20-40 minutes. These essays can be set in a few ways - ranging from those you prepare at home and bring in material for, to those you see for the first time in the exam. They are often based around a midwifery journal or opinion article, or a midwifery centred question.

•The second type is an exam with sentences and questions to complete, to test basic knowledge of language, punctuation and spelling.

You should find out the type of exam so you can target your revision.

Essay Exams

If you have 30 minutes to write an essay, you should write a minimum of 300 words and a maximum of 600, depending on how quickly you can write. It's more important to produce something well-crafted as opposed to something long!

You don't need a really complicated, comprehensive essay. As long as it is **grammatically correct**, the **spelling is mainly correct** (especially basic midwifery terms), it flows well, and doesn't make any mistakes indicating you are not a suitable candidate, it will pass.

Mistakes that might cost you include:

• Misspelling midwife, midwives, midwifery etc.

• Mentioning your experience of caring for a client and writing about them in a way which breaches confidentiality (this is a big deal, don't make this mistake).

• Mentioning you don't want to be a midwife (no really, it's happened).

• Swearing or being unprofessional in any way.

• Meandering in your writing to the point where it doesn't flow.

If you are asked to bring some resources along with you, I would choose no more than 5; perhaps 2 textbooks and 3 journal articles. The textbooks should be chosen for **concise, interesting summaries of the topic** you have been given and the journals should cover several slants on the chosen topic. Have a few key areas or quotes highlighted and prepare how you will use them.

My recommendations for textbooks include:

• Mayes Midwifery

• Myles Midwifery

• The New Midwifery: Science and Sensitivity in Practice

• Midwifery: Best Practice

These textbooks can be expensive to buy - but you can find good, usable chunks of these for free online at 'Google books'! You can use these to prepare for your essay.

The articles should be from journals with good reputations, for instance:

• The Lancet

• The British Journal of Midwifery

• MIDIRS Midwifery Digest

• Journal of Midwifery and Women's Health

• The Practising Midwife

Most of these can also be found online, but local university libraries might help as well.

If you are asked to submit a bibliography or reference list, you can use the following site to teach you how to use Harvard Referencing (which is the most common form of referencing recommended by midwifery lecturers):

education.exeter.ac.uk/dll/studyskills/harvard_refere ncing.htm. If you've been set this kind of essay, you'll be expected to quote or summarise from academic texts. Here's an example:

'Most pregnant women find they need to reduce the amount of exercise they do during the last few months of pregnancy (L.Brown, 1995)'

You can see how to put an entire essay of this nature together in Chapter Seven. It's not hard to get the hang of it, you just make your point or quote as normal and then put the author's name and the year of publication in brackets at the end of the sentence.

Also you should check out the resources I have provided in Chapter Five, page 100 on finding information for your specialist interest subject as they feature good suggestions for researching.

Essay Resources:

www.bbc.co.uk/schools/gcsebitesize/english_literatu re/prosejaneeyre/4prose_janeeyre_sprev1.shtml

www.lifehack.org/articles/communication/7-tips-for-writing-exam-essays.html

Language comprehension resources:

www.bbc.co.uk/bitesize/ks3/english/reading/senten ces/revision/1/

www.bbc.co.uk/skillswise/topic-group/word-grammar

There is also one example of each type of test and sample answers in Chapter Seven.

Why it's so important you prepare well for these extra tests:

Some universities have so many applicants that they use these other selection activities as **screening tools**. This means they do group activities, numeracy and literacy tests as a means of working out who gets to the panel interview section of the selection process. It means you need a pass mark in these tests to get a chance at interviewing for your place as a student midwife. Not all universities do this - but it is essential information for you to know.

But don't panic! If you prepare well there's no reason you can't pass these tests easily.

Use the next chapter to do some practice tests, and you'll be well on your way to becoming a student midwife!

Chapter Seven: Practice Questions And Answers

Practice Numeracy Tests

There are 25 questions in each test. You should restrict yourself to 25 minutes for this test. You need to get 23 correct to pass the test. Remember to include units e.g. mg, ml, seconds, etc. as many universities will mark questions wrong without the correct units.

These tests are designed to be without a calculator, though if your university sets calculator tests, you can of course use one.

Test One

[1]

In your local corner shop there are 2 boxes of tea. One has 160 tea bags and costs £2.99. One has 500 tea bags and costs £7.99. Which is better value?

[2]

If there are 40 patients on the three wards in maternity, and 60% of patients have just one visitor with them, how many patients and visitors do you have altogether on the ward?

[3]

What is 5 x 6 + 14?

[4]

What is the square root of 49?

[5]

A patient of yours has had some painful tightenings this week. She says she has been contracting regularly for 1/8 of Monday, 3/4 of Tuesday, 3/4 of Wednesday, and just 1/16 of Thursday. Work out how many hours in total she has been contracting regularly.

[6]

A 50 kg patient needs some fluids. She should have 3 ml/kg/hour. How much fluid in **litres** will she be given over a 12 hour period?

[7]

What is 36% as its simplest fraction?

[8]

A dietician recommends a patient should lose 10kg to start a new lifestyle. If one kg = 2.2lb, and the patient best understands lb., how many lb. would you tell her to lose?

[9]

A hospital jug holds 3l. It is 4/5 full. How many **ml** is this?

[10]

You are helping design a new area on the ward. You see a scale drawing for the proposed area; it is 4.9 cm in length. The scale is 0.5 cm: 1m. Work out the actual length of the proposed area.

[11]

Round this number to two decimal places: 103.056

[12]

You are using an old fashioned drip set up as all the pumps are busy. There are 50 drops over 1 minute. 20 drop = 1ml. How many hours would it take to administer 150ml?

[13]

A baby is hypothermic (cold) at 36.2 degrees centigrade. You use skin to skin contact to bring the baby's temperature up to an acceptable 37.0 degrees centigrade. How much has the baby's temperature increased by?

[14]

A patient needs drug x to be administered. 30ml of drug x should be mixed in a ratio of 1:100 with IV fluids. How much fluid in ml will this make in total?

[15]

A health board is attempting to increase the number of education classes in their district (see table below). Express the number of people who went to classes in Cambridge Centre as the simplest possible fraction of the total for all four centres.

District	Number of people attending classes 2000-2010
Cambridge Centre	4800
Ely	159
Market Harborough	254
Cambourne	787

[16]

A student diary is for sale in the university bookshop. You remember last year's was £6.00. This year it is £8.01. What percentage has it increased by?

[17]

A nurse has worked between 10.15 and 23.00. She
does this for four days a week. How many minutes
does she work a week?

[18]

A child drinks milk every day. Work out the mean
milk drunk over 4 days based on the table below:

Day	ml of milk
Tuesday	522
Wednesday	250
Thursday	1060
Friday	355

[19]

In a group of 1000 women, the ratio of non-smokers
to smokers is 9:1. How many are smokers and how
many are non-smokers?

[20]

Leanne has been advised to drink no more than 80
ml/hr. over 24 hours. She drinks 2400ml over the
course of 12 hours, and nothing during the 12 hours

overnight. On average, how many ml per hour has
she drunk?

[21]

A patient has lost 5kg and now weighs 195kg. What
percentage of weight has she lost?

[22]

A baby is administered some paracetamol. It needs 15
mg per kg. The baby weighs 4kg. How much
paracetamol should you administer?

[23]

A label states that a medication contains 2.5 mg per
ml of drug. How many mg are in 20 ml?

[24]

A patient needs some insulin. She takes insulin based
on her blood sugar levels. For a week, her needs for
insulin units per day are: 7, 18, 7, 7, 21, 28, 7, 8. What
is the median value of her insulin units needed?

[25]

What is the mode of the insulin units in question 24?

END OF TEST

To mark your work, turn to page 149

Test Two

[1]

A medication has 100mg per ml. A patient needs 1.2 g
of the drug. What is this in ml?

[2]

A patient needs 120mg of a medication per kg. The
patient weighs 50kg. How much medication is
needed?

[3]

A woman has had 5 babies. The babies' weights have
been 3.5 kg, 2.9 kg, 4.0 kg and 3.8 kg. What is the
median weight of her babies?

[4]

A patient measures her glucose values 3 times a day.
Results are in mmol/litre. For three days her values
are: Day one was 5.5, 6.3 and 14. Day two was 3.6,
5.2, 6.3, and day three was 3.9, 7.7, 6.3. What is her
modal value for the three days?

[5]

You see 4 patients during the day. Their weights are:
48 kg, 75 kg, 50 kg and 67 kg. What is the mean
weight in kg?

[6]

A patient has reduced her alcohol intake by 20%. She usually drinks 15 units a week. How many units per week does she drink now?

[7]

A patient has 10 children. 1:5 of these children have colour blindness. What is this as a percentage? How many children have colour blindness?

[8]

A student midwife needs to work 16.5 practice hours. How many shifts starting at 07:15 and finishing at 15:00 does she need to work?

[9]

You are buying a piece of equipment for your unit. One piece of equipment, machine 'A', was £7000, but has been reduced by 8%. The other piece of equipment, machine 'B' is £6095. Which is cheaper?

[10]

The table below expresses what food babies are introduced to first when they are beginning to be weaned (data from a study). Express the number of babies that were given baby rice as their first food as a percentage of the total, and the simplest fraction possible:

Baby Food	Number of babies

Baby Rice	8
Pureed Apple	6
Pureed Carrot	10
Mashed Banana	6

[11]

A drug is mixed with water to be given to a patient. 30 units are given in 500ml water. Give the ratio of units: water.

[12]

A way to convert Celsius to Fahrenheit is to first (*9), then (/5) and then (+32). How much is 20 degrees Celsius in Fahrenheit?

[13]

There is 0.02 mg of drug in every drop of oral medication. A baby needs 0.8 mg. How many drops are needed?

[14]

What is 6 x 9 + 24?

[15]

A birth pool has a 650 litre capacity. It is half full.
How many litres is this?

[16]

A baby weighs 3.2 kg at 5 days. Her birth weight was
3.68 kg. She can lose 10% of her birth weight before a
review and plan needs to be put in place. Does she
need a review and plan?

[17]

What is the fraction 15/25 in its simplest form? What
is this as a percentage?

[18]

A patient needs 4ml/kg/hour of fluids. She weighs
53kg. How much fluid will she need over a 12 hour
period in **litres**?

[19]

A patient is supposed to take an iron tonic every day,
but finds it unpleasant. She needs to take 10ml. On
Monday she takes 1/2 the dose, on Tuesday 3/4, on
Wednesday she manages the whole dose. How many
mls in total has the patient drunk? Round this up to
the nearest whole number and give you answer in ml.

[20]

What is the square root of 64?

[21]

Round this price to the nearest pound: £3.50

[22]

What is 6 + (7 x 22 +3)?

[23]

There are 150 babies born in a month. 60% of them are boys. How many are girls?

[24]

How many ml are in 3/5 of a litre?

[25]

A patient's pulse is 22 over 15 seconds. What is it over 1 minute?

END OF TEST

To mark your work, turn to page 154

Practice Literacy Tests

Type 1: Essays

This question was set in advance of the interview day so candidates could prepare for. However candidates were not allowed to bring in resources on the day.

(You can however see this test as an example of how to use resources in the exam room - you can simply insert references as seen in the section on page 121)

You have thirty minutes to complete this question:

What benefits does exercise provide for pregnant women?

A sample answer and analysis can be found starting on page 159.

Type 2: Language Comprehension

You have 20 minutes to complete this test. I have designed this test to be a fairly challenging example of a language comprehension test. You need to get 10 questions correct to pass.

[1]

Straightaway is an example of a compound word. Please match the words in the first group with a suitable word from the second to make more compound words.

else

basket

sweet

earth

up

spear

quake

ball

meat

where

stream

mint

[2]

Please circle the adverb which is most suitable for the gap in the following sentence:

The teacher .... helped the boy.

kindly

loosely

suspectly

mightily

[3]

Please circle the most suitable word to complete the sentence:

The lady .... the man's shoes.

complemented

complimented

complicated

consecrated

[4]

Please circle the most suitable pronoun to complete the sentence:

.... was cycling in the rain.

Him

They

He

[5]

Please fill in either 'its' or 'it's' in the correct gaps in the sentence:

.... a shame most students do not enjoy grammar
as .... nuances can be quite fun; .... an essential
part of language learning though some of .... rules
can be hard to remember.

[6]

Please fill in either 'bye', 'by' or 'buy' in the correct
gaps in the sentence:

I said .... to my boyfriend and went to .... some
bread; as I did so a small dog walked .... the
window.

[7]

A word in the following sentence is in **bold.** Please
choose an antonym from the list which means the
opposite of the word.

There was a **fragrant** smell coming from the kitchen.

unpleasant

perfumed

savoury

aromatic

[8]

A word in the following sentence is in **bold.** Please
choose an adjective from the list which means the
opposite of the word.

The lady was very **intelligent**.

clever

silly

unintelligent

lazy

[9]

The word below is spelt phonetically. Please write the correct spelling next to the word.

sillabels

[10]

Please add the appropriate punctuation, to the paragraph below, including capital letters:

Labour claimed the proposal was "unravelling" Shadow childrens minister lucy powell told the BBC What the government have announced today is £750m which they say will be shared between £1.9m families - I work that out to be around £400 a year for the average family So they are making this sound a little bit more attractive than it actually is

[11]

Please rewrite the sentences below in the past tense. The verbs in **bold** are the words that needed to be changed.

I **am** hungry today.

It **is** rainy today.

The wind **blows** today.

[12]

Please choose the correct spelling for the following sentence:

The shopping she does is ....

acceptabel

acceptable

acceptible

END OF TEST

To mark your work, turn to page 162.

Practice Panel Interview Questions

You should have a look at the 5 questions every candidate should prepare for, on pages 86-90, as well as looking at the questions below.

These questions cover a large range of topics. I have also included a range of complexities - some questions are very challenging, others are easy or act as a conversation starter between you and the interviewers. All are based on real interview questions.

I would suggest speaking slowly, thinking about your answer and knowing that your ability to answer fact-based or more challenging questions will probably be similar to every other candidate in your position. Do your preparation and then remember:

"Midwives in the making know it - but they also have to show it!"

(Are you bored of me saying it yet?!)

If you are really stuck, be honest and say you don't have enough the information to answer.

You could mention a source where you could get the information - for instance, the Cochrane Library, NICE, or if it's a question about being out in practice, you could say you would ask a qualified midwife for help.

However, after you say all this, make sure you have a stab at an answer which you think might be right.

You'll see what I mean in the answers section, which
also gives analysis of the questions.

A word of warning though - don't just learn all the
answers off by heart! That would be insane as there's
over 50 of them! It would also come across as pretty
odd to your interviewers - at best. At worst they will
recognise plagiarism which might damage your
chances of getting onto a course.

You should use your own experience and knowledge
to prepare. The sample questions and answers should
however give you an idea of what the interviewers will
be looking for and tell you about common errors to
avoid.

In your interview you will almost certainly be asked a
question you haven't prepared for. The trick is not to
panic, but to think it through and offer something
sensible. The DOPE acronym in Chapter Three
might well be helpful.

Your interviewers know that you have not been
trained yet so you will be forgiven easily for not
knowing everything. They just want to see if you can
have a go at all questions with some plausibility, and
whether you seem on a personal level suitable for the
role.

When it comes to questions about you, make sure you
read your personal statement before your interview,
so you can show consistency. Concentrate on the
positive aspects of your personality, experience and
transferable skills; try not to concentrate on things

you aren't so good at. You can identify how you are
improving in some areas, **but your interviewers will
not expect you to be brutally honest about any
shortcomings.**

Questions On Your Personality And How You Will Cope With The Challenges Of The Course

1. What kind of reading have you done around the
subject of midwifery?

2. How do you think you will cope with working
unsocial hours, and with all the course demands?

3. What are you most proud of in your life?

4. If you were struggling academically with a project
or essay at university, how would you address this?
What do you struggle with most academically?

5. Describe how you best fit into a team. What are the
challenges when people try and work in teams?

6. Midwifery can be emotionally demanding. How do
you think you would cope with an unexpected
outcome or stillbirth?

7. Midwifery is a job with massive personal and legal
responsibilities. How do you think you would cope
with this?

8. Describe yourself in three words.

9. How would you cope with difficult situations like being very tired on shift due to unsocial hours?

10. It is difficult sometimes not to feel personally involved or even accountable for a pregnancy loss or adverse event. How would you cope with this type of situation?

11. What do you think were the most important skills to demonstrate in the group discussion?

12. How will this course affect your family and friends?

13. What will your personal coping strategies be for this course?

14. What does the term 'research' mean to you? How would you apply this to an essay you were writing? What about applying research to practice?

15. How do you think you would cope with a degree level course/How do you feel about entering a degree level course at the beginning, as you have completed a degree before?

16. How will you cope financially and socially? You understand placements can start very early in the morning or include on call during the night, how would you cope with this, and have you thought about where you would live?

17. Why do you think this university would suit your needs?

18. What would change your life the most on this course?

19. How would you look after women from a different culture, socio-economic background, or religion from you?

20. If you thought you were excelling at writing an essay and were told you had failed, how would you react?

21. Do you struggle to use computers? Do you have good IT skills?

22. What do you think will be the most rewarding aspect of the job? And the least?

23. How would you cope if a colleague disagreed with you?

24. How would you cope if we did not offer you a place on this occasion?

25. What makes you a better applicant than the other candidates?

26. How would you act as an advocate for women?

27. What do you plan to do within the next 5 years?

28. Are your family supportive of your plans to become a midwife?

29. How would you react to criticism from a qualified midwife which was heard by other students or professionals? How about in front of a client?

30. Was there a specific experience that made you want to be a midwife?

31. How did your work experience prepare you for a role as a midwife?

Sample answers and analysis can be found starting on page 169.

Questions On Your Personal Opinions And Factual Knowledge About Midwifery And Related Topics

1. What do you think midwives do on a day to day basis? What do different types of midwives do?

2. If you were looking after a woman who refused an important part of medical care, how would you approach the subject?

3. What barriers do you think midwives face in inner city areas? What about in rural areas?

4. What kind of other professionals do midwives work with?

5. Midwives are very important in terms of women's health. What benefit do they have on society as a whole?

6. How will you cope counselling or reassuring frightened families or partners? What if their concerns are irrational, for instance, they worry that the baby

isn't getting enough fluid breastfeeding despite
feeding going well?

7. Do you think having had children is an advantage
as a midwife?

8. Why are midwives essential to women's health, as
opposed to having nurses or doctors perform the
same function?

9. Women often have a birth partner with them
during labour. What do you think their role is? How
would you support them through all aspects of
midwifery care?

10. What have you seen in the news recently in terms
of midwifery? How do you think midwives are treated
by the press?

11. What does normal/natural birth mean to you?

12. Do you think it's important midwifery has become
a degree based programme?

13. Imagine you are a woman in labour. What are
your needs? What is most important to you?

14. Breastfeeding can be a contentious issue. Can you
describe some of the benefits and issues?

15. Homebirth can also be a contentious issue. Can
you describe some of the debate? What are your
personal ideas?

16. How would you deal with difficult or aggressive clients or partners/families?

17. What do you think about the rising caesarean rate?

18. Describe why prioritising privacy and dignity for clients is important

19. If you had to prioritise two main attributes a midwife should have, what would they be?

20. Can you list some things you think would **not** take place in a normal labour?

21. What is the biggest change in midwifery within the last forty years?

22. Should we have more male midwives?

Sample answers can be found starting on page 197.

Scenario Based Questions

1. Tell me about different positions women may find useful in labour? What about for giving birth?

2. Jehovah's witness clients have a religious belief that means they will not or cannot accept blood products. How would you react looking after a woman in your care who was dying through this choice?

3. You are looking after a woman with social services input. She has had her first two babies taken into care because of drug use and a violent home. She comes to

see you pregnant with her third child. How would you cope with the situation?

4. How would you cope if a family member of yours commented adversely about a pregnant teenager in public?

5. How would you make women feel comfortable to breastfeed in public, if you had unlimited resources?

A sample answer and analysis can be found starting on page 216.

Answers To Numeracy Tests

You need to get 23 correct to pass the test. Remember to mark units e.g. mg, ml, seconds, etc. as many universities will mark questions wrong without the correct units.

Test One

[1]

Since we don't need an exact answer of the price per tea bag, only the best value option we can do a simple comparison; 160 bags for £3 (rounded up by 1p) is the same as 480 bags for £9 - comparing 480 bags for roughly £9 and 500 bags costing £7.99. We can see that the 500 bag box is better value.

[2]

We need start by finding out what 60% of 40 is.

1% of 40 = 0.4 (because 40/100 = 0.4)

0.4 x 60 = 60%

0.4 x 60 = 24

So there are 24 visitors.

24 visitors + 40 patients = 64 patients and visitors all together

[3]

Using BODMAS, ((5 x 6) + 14) = (30 + 14) = 44

[4]

7 x 7 = 49, therefore the answer is 7.

[5]

1/8 of Monday = 1/8 of 24 hrs = 24/8 = 3 hours. 3/4 of Tuesday = 3/4 of 24 hours = 24/4 x 3 = 6 x 3 = 18 hours. The same for Wednesday.1/16 of Thursday = 1/16 of 24 hours = 24/16 which to simplify by halving = 12/8 = 6/4 = 3/2. 3/2 = 1.5. Therefore 1.5 hours. The total number of hours added together = 40.5

[6]

50 x 3 = 150. 150 x 12 = (150 x 10 = 1500) + (150 x 2 = 300) = 1800 ml = 1.8 litres

[7]

36/100 = (/2) 18/50 = (/2) 9/25

[8]

1 kg = 2.2lb. 10 x 2.2 = 22. Therefore 10kg = 22lb.

[9]

3 l = 3000ml. 3000/5= 600. 4 x 600 = 2400 ml

[10]

4.9/0.5 = estimate = 5.0/0.5 = 10m ish. 4.9/0.5 = 49/5 = 9 with 4 remaining. 9 into 40 = 8. Therefore 4.9/0.5 = 9.8m

[11]

103.06, as the unit in bold is over 5: 103.05**6**

[12]

20 drops = 1 ml. (/2) 10 drops = 0.5ml. (/10) 1 drop = 0.05ml.

150/0.05 = easier to work out 150/0.5 = 300 drops. x 10 to account for 0.05 = 3000 drops. 3000/50 = 300/5 = 60 minutes.

Overall, 1 hour.

[13]

0.8 degrees centigrade

[14]

1:100 = 30: (100 x 30)= 3000. = 30:3000. 30 + 3000 = 3030 ml

[15]

A health board is attempting to increase the number of education classes in their district (see table below). Express the number of people who went to classes in Cambridge Centre as the simplest possible fraction of the total for all four centres.

District	Number of people attending classes 2000-2010
Cambridge Centre	4800
Ely	159
Market Harborough	254
Cambourne	787

$4800 + 159 + 254 + 787 = 6000$

$4800/6000 = 48/60$ (if you divide by 10)

$48/60 = 8/10$ (if you divide by 6)

$8/10 = 4/5$ (if you divide by 2)

4/5 is the answer because there are no more lowest common denominators

[16]

6.00 = 100%. 8.01 - 6.00 = 2.01. An estimation = £2 increase. 2/6 = 1/3 = 33%. 2.01/6 = ?/100.

2.01/6 = 03.35 x 100

= 33.5% increase.

[17]

10.15 to 23.00 = 12 hours and 45 minutes. 12 hours 45 minutes, in minutes = (12 x 60) + 45 = 720 + 45 = 765 minutes per day. 765 x 4 = 3060 minutes a week.

[18]

522 + 250 + 1060 + 355 = 2187. 2187/4 = 546.75

[19]

9 +1 = 10 parts expressed altogether.

1000/10 = 100

If 100 are smokers then 900 are non smokers.

[20]

2400/24 = 100 ml/hour

[21]

A patient has lost 5kg and now weighs 195kg. What percentage of weight has she lost?

195+5kg = old weight or 200 kg = 100%

So if each kg represents 0.5% then 5 kg = the patient lost 2.5%

[22]

15 x 4 = 60 mg

[23]

2.5 x 20 = 50mg

[24]

7, 7, 7, 7, 8, 18, 21, 28 = (7+8)/2 = 7.5 units

[25]

(Modal average is the most common value that appears in a set of data) = 7 units

Test Two

You need to get 23 correct to pass the test. Remember to mark units e.g. mg, ml, seconds, etc. as many universities will mark questions wrong without the correct units.

[1]

100 mg per ml = 0.1 g per 1 ml

0.1 x 12 = 1.2g

1 ml x 12 = 12ml

[2]

50 x 120 = (100 x 120 = 12000)/2 = 6000mg

[3]

In order: 2.9, 3.5, 3.8, 4.0

$3.5 + 3.8 = 7.3$

$7.3/2 = 3.65$kg

[4]

In order: 3.6, 3.9, 5.2, 5.5, 6.3, 6.3, 6.3, 7.7, 14

Mode = the most frequent number 6.3

6.3 mmol/litre

[5]

$48 + 75 + 50 + 67 = 241$

Mean $= 240/4 = (240/2 = 120)/2 = 60$ kg

[6]

15 units = 100%. $15/100 * 20 = 3$. $15 - 3 = 12$ units

[7]

The question is asking for a conversion of the ratio 1:5 into a percentage which is 20%, then 20% of 10 = 2 children.

[8]

A student midwife needs to work 16.5 practice hours. How many shifts starting at 07:15 and finishing at 15:00 does she need to work?

07:15 to 15:00 = 8hrs 15mins or 8.25 hrs
$16.5/8.25 = 2$

The student midwife must complete 2 more shifts.

[9]

For this question an exact calculation is not necessary.

10% of 7000 is 700. So if machine 'A' was reduced by 10 it would cost £6300, which is more that machine 'B' which costs £6095.

[10]

$8+6+10+6 = 30$
$8/30 = 4/15$

[11]

$30:500 = 3:50$

[12]

$20*9 = 180$
$180/5 = 36$

$36+32 = 68$

[13]

$0.8/0.02 =$ (to simplify) $= 80/2 = 40$
40 drops are needed to administer 0.8mg

[14]

$6*9 = 54$
$54 + 24 = 78$

[15]

$650/2 = 325$ litres

[16]

3.68 / 10 = 0.368
3.680 - 0.368 = 3.312
Yes, the baby does need a review.

[17]

1/5 = 0.2 %

x by 3 to find:

3/5 = 0.6%

15/40 = 15/40

[18]

4*53 = 212

212*10 = 2120
212*2 = 424
2120 + 424 = 2544 mls

= 2.544 litres

[19]

Monday = 10*.5 = 5
Tuesday = 10*.75 = 7.5
Wednesday = 10
10 + 7.5 + 5 = 23ml

[20]

8*8 = 64
The square root is 8

[21]

£4.00 (The question was round £3.50 to the nearest pound…if you are asked to round up a number which falls exactly half way between the applicable integers (in this case whole pounds), you always round up.

[22]

7 x 22 = 154
154 + 3 = 157
157 + 6 = 163

[23]

There are 150 babies born in a month. 60% of them are boys. How many are girls?

40% are girls
40/100 x 150 = 60 girls

[24]

⅗ = 6/10 = 60%
60% of 1,000ml is 600ml
There are 600 ml in ⅗ of a litre.

[25]

15*4 = 60s = 1 minute
22*4 = 88
The patients pulse is 88 beats per minute.

Answers To Literacy Tests

Type 1: Essays

You have thirty minutes to complete this question:

What benefits does exercise provide for pregnant women?

Mind mapping the question revealed these possible topics to write about:

• Weight gain: lack of ability to move in labour; long term health concerns

• Pre-eclampsia; some suggestion that exercise can make a difference in pre-eclampsia

• Mood: depression is on the rise and pregnancy can be a worrying time; it can also be a social connection; it can also be very important in balancing life and introducing children to exercise

• Problems overheating: fainting is more likely due to the pregnancy hormones; there is some evidence of birth defects

Planning your structure:

Around 60 words minimum is needed for each topic, leaving 100 words or so for introduction and conclusion.

Example essay answer:

Exercise at any time of life is recommended for a
multitude of reasons. It is enjoyable, healthy, and
there is evidence to suggest it has particular benefits
in pregnancy.

Weight gain can be a problem in pregnancy, and
exercise can help address this. Obesity is a problem in
society generally and some women, for lots of reasons
outside the scope of this essay, can put on weight in
pregnancy. Exercise should be encouraged to build
muscle which increases basal metabolic rate, therefore
avoiding obesity. This is important in pregnancy as
obesity can reduce the ability to move or employ
helpful techniques like labouring upright or in the
birth pool. Obesity can also cause long term health
concerns like diabetes, heart disease and all of the
other known complications.

There is some evidence to suggest exercise also can
impact pre-eclampsia, the difficult-to-control
condition which can occur in some pregnancies. Pre-
eclampsia is an unpleasant condition and can end in
premature iatrogenic delivery of babies; there is, in
some cases, no other option. If exercise has a positive
effect on pre-eclampsia, it could be a cheap way of
combating the disorder which also has other health
benefits.

In some cases depression can be controlled with
exercise. Though avoiding or stopping
antidepressants must be looked at by a physician on a
case by case basis, antidepressants can have an

adverse effect on some pregnancies. Therefore exercise could be an excellent alternative. Mild depression that does not need medication could be eliminated through exercise. It can also be a healthy part of adapting to be a new parent - it can be a social activity, for instance, walking with other mothers who like to take their babies out. This also has benefits for the children of these pregnancies, as they will be introduced to exercise early in life, and to a social group of their peers.

A feared aspect of exercise for pregnant women and some practitioners is overheating. Due to hormonal changes, fainting is more likely for some women when pregnant. Overheating can lead to this, and could possibly lead to a fall, which could have bad consequences. There is evidence to suggest birth defects can occur if a foetus is exposed to high temperatures too often. For these reasons exercise should not be too strenuous. If a woman is feeling pain, is breathless to the point where she can't hold a normal conversation, or feeling dizzy, then she should stop.

In conclusion, exercising in pregnancy has more benefits than negative aspects. It should be a practice all the way through life to address physical and mental fitness. It should however be done with some caution to control any side effects like birth defects or simple dizziness.

This answer would achieve high marks as:

• The work was between 300 - 600 words.

• The writing flows well with a clear structure; it uses a 'point - example - explain' format most of the way through which helps the reader navigate through the essay.

• There are no spelling mistakes, especially in relation to midwifery.

• There are both simple and complex sentences.

• Punctuation is used correctly throughout the piece.

Type 2: Language Comprehension

You had 20 minutes to complete your test. You need to get 10 questions correct to pass.

[1]

Straightaway is an example of a compound word. Please match the words in the first group with the suitable second the make further compound words.

else

basket

sweet

earth

up

spear

quake

ball

meat

where

stream

mint

elsewhere

basketball

sweetmeat

earthquake

upstream

spearmint

[2]

Please underline the adverb from the list which is most suitable for the gap in the following sentence:

The teacher .... helped the boy.

<u>kindly</u>

loosely

suspectly

mightily

[3]

Please underline the most suitable word from the list
to complete the sentence:

The lady .... the man's shoes.

complemented

<u>complimented</u>

complicated

consecrated

[4]

Please circle the most suitable pronoun to complete
the sentence:

.... was cycling in the rain.

Him

They

<u>He</u>

[5]

Please fill in either 'its' or 'it's' in the correct gaps in
the sentence:

.... a shame most students do not enjoy grammar as .... nuances can be quite fun; .... an essential part of language learning though some of .... rules can be hard to remember.

It's a shame most students do not enjoy grammar as **its** nuances can be quite fun; **it's** an essential part of language learning though some of **its** rules can be hard to remember.

[6]

Please fill in either ' 'bye' or 'by' or 'buy' in the correct gaps in the sentence:

I said .... to my boyfriend and went to ...... some bread; as I did so a small dog walked .... the window.

I said **bye** to my boyfriend and went to **buy** some bread; as I did so a small dog walked **by** the window.

[7]

A word in the following sentence is in **bold.** Please underline an antonym from the list which means the opposite of the word.

There was a **fragrant** smell coming from the kitchen.

perfumed

<u>unpleasant</u>

savoury

aromatic

[8]

A word in the following sentence is in **bold.** Please underline an adjective from the list which means the opposite of the word.

The lady was very **intelligent.**

silly

clever

<u>unintelligent</u>

lazy

[9]

The word below is spelt phonetically. Please write the correct spelling under the word.

sillabels

correct spelling: syllables

[10]

Please add the appropriate punctuation, to the paragraph below, including capital letters:

Labour claimed the proposal was "unravelling" Shadow childrens minister lucy powell told the BBC What the government have announced today is £750m which they say will be shared between £1.9m families - I work that out to be around £400 a year for the average family So they are making this sound a little bit more attractive than it actually is

With appropriate punctuation:

Labour claimed the proposal was "unravelling". Shadow children's minister Lucy Powell told the BBC: 'What the government have announced today is £750m, which they say will be shared between 1.9m families. I work that out to be around £400 a year for the average family, so they are making this sound a little bit more attractive than it actually is'.

(If your answer looks something like this you are likely to pass - it doesn't have to be identical, as long as your punctuation and use of capital letters is correct).

[11]

Please rewrite the sentences below in the past tense. The verbs in **bold** are the words that needed to be changed.

I **am** hungry today.

It **is** rainy today.

The wind **blows** today.

I **was** hungry today.

It **was** rainy today

The wind **blew** today.

[12]

Please underline the correct spelling for the following
sentence:

The shopping she does is ....

acceptabel

<u>acceptable</u>

acceptible

Practice Panel Interview Answers

Analysis of the questions is provided in italics. My
sample answers follow. Hopefully this will aid you to
prepare your own answers and technique - reciting
answers will almost certainly be obvious and
unconvincing, and do you no favours, but it is often
helpful to see sample answers to put the interview in
context and avoid common mistakes.

When reading this section, please remember I am a
qualified midwife and I wrote these answers under
'armchair conditions'! Don't be put off if they seem
very comprehensive, you don't have to answer every
questions perfectly! Just use them as your inspiration
and for information.

Analysis And Sample Answers: On Your Personality And How You Will Cope With The Challenges Of The Course

1. What kind of reading have you done around the subject of midwifery?

*This question is asking how much enthusiasm you have for the
subject, how much academic insight you have, and if you have a
specialist area of interest.*

I have done quite a bit of interesting reading.
Textbooks offer a good overview and I have dipped
in and out of Mayes midwifery and Myles midwifery

textbooks. Spiritual midwifery by Ina May Gaskin also
gives a bit of political information and I really like her
basic guide to physiology.

In terms of journals, I like to look at the MIDIRS
journal, Midwifery Today and a few others. The
Lancet has some good information as well. I like to
follow back research from Cochrane trials - for
instance, the British Journal of Midwifery published
an article recently on waterbirth in England and Wales
and basically the conclusion was there seemed to be
no adverse outcomes but there is still more data
needed. The interesting thing is the House of
Commons is quoted in the introduction and they
recommended, even with the limited amount of data
available, that every woman should have the option of
a birthing pool if practicable. Obviously there's lots of
politics involved in birth and sometimes they trump
the evidence base (though in this case I thoroughly
approve of the outcome of more birth pools!)

2. How do you think you will cope with working unsocial hours, and with all the course demands?

*This question is trying to find the candidates who won't cope
with difficult hours. Even if you are not quite sure how you will
work this out, it is better to reassure your interviewers at this
point; they are merely trying to work out if you are truly
unsuited to the midwifery lifestyle. This question is also asking
if you have a realistic idea of the demands of the course.*

I've worked shifts in my work experience and saw it
as a bit of a trial run. It was fine. I'm used to working
around lots of different schedules - this is just life! My

partner and I use an online diary to work out quality time, job time, study time etc. I also try to get the basics right when working night shifts, so sleep, food and a bit of exercise. I think I've got a very realistic idea of how many hours I will need to put in.

In terms of the course demands, I have coped with a demanding academic diary this year, along with a part time job and looking after my sister's children (which will be something that changes if I start training). I like a challenge - I think it's important to have time off, to keep interested in what you're doing and not burn out - but I work best when challenged.

3. What are you most proud of in your life?

This question is really assessing your ability to think fast and choose something true about your life that you are proud of that has transferable skills to midwifery! Therefore, instead of saying something like, 'I'm most proud of my ability to cook a really amazing dinner party ending with a pavlova,' it's probably better to say something like:

I have a good circle of friends who I have known for years. We meet at least once a month and generally have a meal and talk about everything from relationships, to work, to children (with one overseas who talks to us on Skype!). I am very proud to be friends with such an amazing group; I've known them from childhood and I benefit so much from their insights. So, my personal relationships are something I am very proud of.

**4. If you were struggling academically with a
project or essay at university, how would you
address this? What do you struggle with most
academically?**

*This question is self-evident - it's trying to screen for students
who are less academically able or those who will struggle without
knowing how to get help and succeed.*

I've been in this position before. A-levels are quite a
step up from GCSEs. I found this especially with
history GCSE to Classical Studies. I really struggled to
get good marks in my first month of college. So I
accessed a few of my college's extra courses on how
to write academic essays, and put together a plan with
my tutor that played to my strengths in terms of
essays (I've always been good at finding an interesting
slant on topics), and addressed my weaknesses of
structure and grammar. This was a big lesson for me;
I now feel very comfortable writing essays for
coursework and under time pressure, and receive
good marks.

So I would imagine most students will find something
challenging academically when studying midwifery
and I would ask for help from the university and
construct a plan, and try to see it as a good way of
improving. I wouldn't say I have any one area of
academic weakness, but I suppose I'm slightly better
at contributing in class than writing essays, although I
now consider myself reasonably strong in both areas.

5. Describe how you best fit into a team. What are the challenges when people try and work in teams?

This question assesses how you will fit in as a midwife/student midwife on the 'shop floor' of wards or community practices. It's trying to ascertain if you will manage to contribute effectively when you are working looking after women in a variety of settings. The interviewers might also be wondering how you will fit in with your student peer group to aid learning.

I am personally the team member that likes to get to the truth of matters. I enjoy researching, and applying evidence to situations. I like to communicate my ideas. I can act as a leader, and as a supporter/follower (I do this in my hobby of rock climbing all the time) but I prefer to be conversing, assessing and applying information. I do not particularly enjoy conflict, but can manage it if required.

Working in teams is so very important in terms of offering a good service - it's ideal if everyone can identify and play to their strengths, while acknowledging and working with other team members' strengths and weaknesses. I expect midwives face these challenges just like any other team of people. I think the advantage midwives have is that presumably everyone wants the same thing: to provide good maternity care for women. So it would be about using that motivation to work with our team's strengths and weaknesses.

6. Midwifery can be emotionally demanding. How do you think you would cope with an unexpected outcome or stillbirth?

This question is trying to see if you would have an appropriate response in these situations. It is also trying to measure your level of maturity and ability to talk about these very difficult topics. I have included two different answers; the first is from the point of view of someone who has never experienced pregnancy loss. The second is from someone who has personal experience.

A] I have never come across this situation before, so the truth is I don't know how I'll react. I have thought about whether I'll be able to cope as obviously it's an essential part of the job - I suspect I'd try very hard to support the woman and her family, using all the resources I had at my command and that any mentors suggest. I would show I was sad in front of the client and her family, but make sure the care was about her grief, not mine. I would also try and talk with mentors or supervisors at an appropriate point to debrief, and I'm sure I would feel very sad and need to have a cry and a think about everything. However, I do think midwives have a really important job to do in these cases and can make even this very sad time in someone's life a little easier.

B] I have personal experience of pregnancy loss, as my mother had a term stillbirth when I was 16. The care she received was very good. I would try to work out how the woman in question and her family wanted to be treated - some women must have specific religious needs, for instance. Others might not know how to react. I'd try and listen really well to their needs and suggest ways of processing the loss, if it seemed like it would help, for instance my family really benefitted from having some professional photos taken of us all together with our baby.

I'm not sure I'd mention my own loss as it's very personal and it might affect the client's grief. However some people might benefit from feeling like they are not the only one - I'd really try and feel my way through with all the resources available, and obviously take the lead from the midwife I was working with.

I'd have a chat with my family, as we are very close and we talk about our loss on a regular basis, which for us is very helpful. Obviously I wouldn't talk about any personal details or betray client confidentiality, though.

7. Midwifery is a job with massive personal and legal responsibilities. How do you think you would cope with this?

This question is trying to assess how you will deal with all the stress involved in midwifery. It's also checking you have a realistic idea of what the job entails.

Midwifery is a fascinating job because it covers care to do with pregnancy, birth and the postnatal period. These are such important times for women - ask any woman of my grandmother's age what their biggest life experience or biggest achievement is and they often say 'having my children'. As it is so important

for women, and substandard care has such massive
consequences on lives, of course it has huge legal and
personal responsibilities. I would try and see it this
way; if you have the privilege and advantage of
looking after people at this point in their lives, the flip
side of this is the responsibility. You can't have one
without the other.

I would try to be a good clinical practitioner, with a
realistic idea of the stresses involved, but I would also
try to never to lose my joy at helping women through
pregnancy and into parenthood.

8. Describe yourself in three words.

*This question doesn't tell your interviewer much even if
answered well. It looks at your ability to think fast and present
them with characteristics you think will be received favourably.
It's worth noting here that if you can't work out why the
interviewer is asking something, it might be simply not a good
question from them! In these situations all you can do is present
some characteristics that they will be looking for in candidates.*

I am interested, motivated and calm. I feel student
midwives need these characteristics so I hope my
personality will be suitable for the role.

9. How would you cope with difficult situations like being very tired on shift due to unsocial hours?

*This is trying to ascertain your suitability to work shifts for
most of your career. Will you be one of the many who drop out
because of the difficult working hours?*

I'm sure everyone has days at work where they are tired, and I'm no different, but I am naturally quite conscientious, so I'd try very hard not to let it impact on being a student midwife. I'd spend more time checking work to make sure it was safe and correct, and perhaps get colleagues I trusted to check one or two things if I was unsure.

I've worked shifts before and I think the key thing is to keep yourself in good condition. So sleep, exercise and time off will be essential around shifts.

10. It is difficult sometimes not to feel personally involved or even accountable for a pregnancy loss or adverse event. How would you cope with this type of situation?

This question is really seeing if you are likely to go to pieces under pressure. It's also seeing if you are able to keep professional distance from the emotional nature of the job.

This would be very hard, and you've posed a difficult question! However I can see how it would be essential to keep your 'game face' on in a situation where a client blamed you for something, or when you felt you had made a mistake in one room, and had to keep going the rest of the shift.

I think pride in your work is essential, but pride can also be quite a dangerous characteristic. If you are so proud of your ability as a midwife that you think you can't make a mistake, I can see how you would feel personally accountable if something went wrong. So I'd try and keep a realistic idea of my abilities, while

keeping my care as conscientious as possible. I'd also
try to keep it in mind that it's natural to blame
yourself when something bad happens, but that this
attitude is often not helpful. Calm, logical, empathetic
care would be better.

11. What do you think were the most important skills to demonstrate in the group discussion?

*Most candidates find it hard to work out what is needed in a
group interview setting...but you know from Chapter Six what
the interviewers are looking for:*

I think you were looking for people to demonstrate
their communication, leadership, negotiation and
teamwork skills. I think anyone dominating the
situation wouldn't have shown good ability. Anyone
not contributing wouldn't have done well either.
Contributing something well thought out in a
confident manner, with the ability to get people to
listen, as well as being able to listen and work with
others were the essentials. These skills are needed in
group situations so are essential skills for midwives.

12. How will this course affect your family and friends?

*This question is again trying to screen for students who will
drop out as the course is very demanding. It also checks you
have a realistic idea of the course demands.*

Well, I won't have as much time to see them, so that's
a downside. But I am used to juggling quite a full
calendar, and my partner is also a professional.

I would need them for support and they are very
happy I've found a career path which I find
fascinating. I work full time at the moment, and have
worked shifts before, so I imagine when I am
qualified it won't be so different from now. During
training I think I'll just have to remind them it's only
for 3 years, and I have to say that so far they've been
extremely supportive! And perhaps if the odd person
was not supportive it would show they weren't a very
good friend!

I plan to continue rock climbing with friends and
family as it will be a useful wind down.

13. What will your personal coping strategies be for this course?

*This question is similar to the last - it is asking how you will
cope with demands on your time and on your emotions, and
your ability to deal with criticism.*

I know midwifery is very demanding in many ways. I
have had demanding jobs combined with life
challenges before - to start I like to get the basics right
if at all possible, with good sleep, food and exercise.
This doesn't have to be too time consuming, it just
means you start with a body and mind that have
major needs satisfied.

I try to act 'deliberately' in stressful situations. It can
be very tempting to let adrenaline make decisions for
you, but I would try and spend a bit of time on
planning activities each week. I like to-do lists and use
an online calendar to plan my time.

I would try to maintain good support with other students, midwives and see my friends and family often. I know I bang on about it all the time, but I find whatever mood I'm in, even a 15 minute rock climb works wonders for my problem solving skills and emotional wellbeing. My partner is also very good at supporting me when I'm challenged or upset. It's just occurred to me that I might be able to make new friends on the course and perhaps they would enjoy climbing - then we could support each other really well!

14. What does the term 'research' mean to you? How would you apply this to an essay you were writing? What about applying research to practice?

This question is trying to work out if you know what research is - many fall into the trap of thinking 'research' is when you go to the library, have a look in books, and use the computer to print out articles. Research is actually an academic term meaning to systematically investigate, and usually will involve either statistical or academic interpretation of results. I have included quite a long, comprehensive answer here which you can abbreviate as you see fit, but do make sure you get the basics across that research is about generating evidence-based conclusions.

Research to me means a few different things. I understand the basics though it is quite complicated: research can be quantitative, which means looking at data to measure it, usually numerically, or qualitative which means looking at various themes or accounts

within a topic. It is a way of investigating topics to
generate evidence-based conclusions.

This means I put my trust into well designed research
trials. It also means, however, that I don't necessarily
believe everything I read in a study or journal article,
because research can be really poorly conducted. It is
also important to remember that research evidence is
sometimes replaced by more up to date information.

So research is very important in midwifery to offer
good, evidence-based care. But it is also important to
recognise its limitations, apply common sense and all
the other crucial aspects of care like personal choice.

**15. How do you think you would cope with a
degree level course? or, How do you feel about
entering a degree level course at the beginning,
as you have completed a degree before?**

*This question is trying to understand what your attitude to
university life might be. It is also trying to work out whether
you will cope academically, or whether you might find the course
unstimulating if you have already studied at degree level. I have
included two examples to cover both options.*

A] I am very excited about a degree level course. I
have recently completed my A-levels and I like
learning; midwifery is a topic that I could read about
all day! I have in the past had some challenges getting
to grips with A-level material, but I think an essential
part of this process has been 'learning to learn'. I now
feel I am equipped to find information to support
myself if I find I'm struggling. So that's been the main

benefit of doing A-levels, and though I struggled to begin with, I am now academically strong.

B] Midwifery is a different subject, I don't expect to be bored! I find midwifery fascinating. If I cope well academically because I have done a degree course before, that's great, and there are plenty of other good ways to occupy any spare time and energy.

16. How will you cope financially and socially? You understand placements can start very early in the morning or include being on call during the night, how would you cope with this, and have you thought about where you will live?

This question is trying to see how much you have researched the practicalities of the course. It is also trying to see if you are worried about any particular area, or if you are unsuitable in another less obvious way.

Financially I understand there is some funding available for course fees and a bursary for many students. I will also strongly consider a student loan, which I know is the best way to borrow money if necessary in my position. It is obviously a step down from my pay at the moment, but I think if anything it proves how committed I am to being a midwife. I am able to plan and budget financially, and just like any student, I see it as an investment in my future.

Socially I plan to keep up with friends and family. I also plan to use my main recreation, rock climbing, to wind down from the pressures of the course, and this is a very social activity. My friends and family are

happy to see me so motivated and interested by a
career prospect!

I do understand that midwifery, as a job, comes with
unsocial hours. I would try very hard to maintain my
wellbeing through healthy diet, adequate exercise and
sleep - I'm a fan of having little naps if I've been up at
odd hours! I also hear from friends who are midwives
that some lovely births come at night, so that's
something to look forward to.

I plan to live locally as I don't want big commutes
around anti-social working hours. I'm not sure about
Uni Halls - I think I'd rather flat share.

17. Why do you think this university would suit your needs?

*This question is trying to see if you have researched the
university you are applying to. It is a good way for interviewers
to find candidates who are likely to excel on their particular
university course.*

*You should research each university and find a targeted answer
for this question.*

I think Leicester would be an excellent place to train
as a midwife. I come from Cambridge originally, and
could apply for the course there, but I think the
clients are not as diverse as in Leicester. It offers a
range of clients with different cultures,
socioeconomic backgrounds, nationalities and
religions. I am also very interested in your resources;
the university here has a reputation for vocational
degrees with an emphasis on doing things 'in the real

world', which is a good attitude for midwifery training
to be based around.

I also think the social side of things looks very good
here - there is an active rock climbing group which I'd
love to get into!

18. What would change your life the most on this course?

*This question again assesses your knowledge of the course
demands, and also tries to dig a little deeper into your
personality and life.*

I have never had this kind of responsibility before -
that appears to be the most life changing thing about
midwifery. It's a bit daunting, but I'm really looking
forward to the work itself, should I get onto the
course.

I have thought about the responsibility aspect of the
job and came to the conclusion that if you want the
privilege of looking after childbearing women, you
have to accept the responsibility.

19. How would you look after women from a different culture, socio-economic background, or religion from you?

*This question is trying to identify any candidates who will have
difficulty looking after a particular set of women. It is also
checking your aptitude for the job; having an appetite for
working with a wide range of people is essential.*

I actually find this exciting. It's part of why I imagine
midwifery doesn't get boring, as you see different

kinds of people every day. It's one of the reasons why
I want to train in a big diverse city instead of
somewhere small. If you're asking how I would react
to working with someone with completely different
life choices and values to me, I would spend time
listening to them actively, trying to work out how I
could best adapt my care to them. I'd try to see it as a
learning process - and sure, some women might have
attributes that were so different to mine I couldn't
really understand, but this is a life challenge not just
specific to midwifery - I'd just keep trying!

**20. If you had done a brilliant job writing an
essay and were told you had failed the paper, how
would you react?**

*This question is trying to see how you would cope with academic
challenges or failures, and if you are able to keep trying even
when things gets tough.*

I would be disappointed of course, but failure is part
of learning. That sounds very lofty - but I've never
mastered anything without having a bit of failure. I
would get some advice from a tutor and try to work
out what went wrong. Hopefully I would make some
progress and get better at writing essays for the next
time I was set one. I think it's important not to take
yourself too seriously, and also to remember that
most students struggle with something at university.

**21. Do you struggle to use computers? Do you
have good IT skills?**

Midwifery requires a basic grasp of how to use a computer for looking up results, recording data and so on. Your interviewers will also be trying to work out if you will be able to access all the information you need for course projects, essays and assessments. These are very basic computer skills almost everyone will pick up fast - you can reassure the interviewers you can cope. I have included two answers to cover those with excellent IT skills and those who have basic skills.

A] No, I have excellent IT skills. I have been researching and doing projects using online resources and using word processors and other pieces of software for a long time. I would say I have a better than average grasp of how to fix computers as well, as my father encouraged us to use computers from a young age.

B] Although sometimes I find it difficult to use certain programs to begin with, I can use word processing software, search online, use cut and paste functions and keep files in order. I can adapt to most things expected of me.

22. What do you think will be the most rewarding aspect of the job? And the least?

*This question is trying to delve into your personal strengths and weaknesses. It's also trying to see if you have a personality which is a good fit for midwifery. Try to avoid talking about superficial aspects of midwifery - for instance, cuddling babies, or cleaning up blood and vomit. The question is asking for the **most** and **least** rewarding aspects of the job. Offer your interviewer something which shows your depth and suitability as a candidate.*

I look forward to helping women achieve something out of their birth plan, or helping them get a particular aspect of their care right for them. I also look forward to making a difference to someone's experience of new parenthood - I read on a midwifery blog that a midwife used a translator with a woman with complex needs from India, and the woman in question had felt strong enough to breastfeed against her parents' wishes, and was really enjoying the experience and happy about providing such good nutrition for her baby. For me it will be the moments when you can empower women that will seem very rewarding. I think all prospective midwives look forward to experience with labour and birth as well!

The least rewarding aspects I'm sure will involve sleep deprivation, spending a long time doing paperwork, and coping with time pressure.

23. How would you cope if a colleague disagreed with you?

This is checking your ability to cope with conflict professionally.

It depends on the situation. I would try to listen to their concerns, properly listening to try and see it from their point of view. If they had more information than me or a better slant on things, I'd be perfectly happy to change my opinions.

However, they might have a different agenda. For instance, if they had a particular personal objection to waterbirth, I would either try to present the information for them and encourage them to think

logically about the situation in a polite way, or thank
them for their opinion and remind them care comes
down to client choice and the evidence base. I would
also remind them that I would support them in their
care of clients if the situation were reversed.

In some situations, conflict can arise. I imagine this is
the case is a maternity care setting just like any other.
If a colleague was speaking angrily or inappropriately
I would proceed as I have just described, but I might
have a trusted colleague or manager listening. If it
turned into a real argument (which wouldn't be
appropriate at work) I would make sure I stayed very
calm and firm, and would ask for a manager to
mediate the situation. I would try to resolve things on
a good note and remind them that everyone needs to
be challenged from time to time, but in this case we
might have to agree to disagree.

24. How would you cope if we did not offer you a place on this occasion?

*This question measures how much you want the role - the
interviewers might really be asking if you are applying on a
whim, or would apply again next year as you are really
committed to becoming a midwife. It might also be a standard
question they are asking to try and offer places to candidates
who really want a place at their specific university. All in all,
quite a tricky question to answer. I would hint at your
likelihood of being offered a place by a different university and
being a good catch, while emphasising their university is your
first choice.*

I would be disappointed as (name of university) is my top choice, because of the city, the demographic of clients, and the diverse placements offered. I also hear there's a really interesting homebirth scheme which is something I'd love to see in action, and perhaps one day if I am lucky enough to be a trained midwife, get involved in.

I have applied to other universities as I am very serious about pursuing this career path. Although I definitely would apply next year for a place as a student midwife, I would much prefer to start this year.

25. What makes you a better applicant than the other candidates?

This can often be a hard question for candidates to answer - you will probably have spent all morning with a group of others, and as you are applying to be a midwife, it's likely you are a kind and empathetic person who doesn't want to be unpleasant! The interviewers are not asking to criticise your contemporaries - what they are really asking here is 'why are you an outstanding candidate?'

Feel free to impress them. List all your attributes, transferrable skills, thinking you have done about the role, and other positives. I'll give two examples, one from candidate who had just left college, one from a mature student who has children.

A] I'm just out of college and I feel strong academically. I have a good idea of what will be demanded of me academically and believe I can cope and even excel in some areas. I am also able to devote

a lot of time and energy to midwifery as I don't have
many family responsibilities yet. For my age I am very
mature, and I have friends and family who are
midwives so I think I know what it entails.

I have spent time researching the job and what it will
be like day to day. I have gone through the National
Childbirth Trust and talked to service users, for
instance a blind mother, a mother who has
experienced a molar pregnancy, a teenage mother, a
black mother and a mother who had been extremely
unwell with pre-eclampsia. I was very interested in
what these women had to say and felt helping with
their care would be a very beneficial and satisfying job
to do.

I get fired up by midwifery as a subject. I've never
spent time flicking through textbooks or looking at
research for fun before. I really think given the tools
and training I can sustainably be a good practitioner
who acts as an advocate for women, and tries to
empower them during their pathway into parenthood.
I am also able to pick up skills quite quickly, and I am
very organised!

I am not applying just because 'I like babies'. I can see
how much work and responsibility is attached, but I
think being a midwife is so much more worthwhile
than working in an office or just to make money. So
for all these reasons I think I am an excellent
candidate, above and beyond other candidates.

B] My personal strengths lie in having a challenging
job that helps empower people. In particular I find

the care of women and their journey into motherhood fascinating and of massive importance to society in general.

I have taken my time to come to the conclusion I would make a good midwife - I have done lots of reading, built up personal friendships with midwives in my social group who are happy to discuss the pros and cons of the job, and had discussions with service users, some of whom were happy with their care, others who could see room for improvement. I think I have a very realistic idea of what I would be doing day to day.

In recent years I've combined this with a love of learning - I think my common sense and ability now to critique research and information in textbooks and journals makes me quite a well-rounded candidate. I have had to get good at academic study and writing in my recent access course, and it's something I've really relished as an adult in a way that I couldn't have achieved just out of school.

I don't think I could ever lose my wonder at pregnancy and birth. You probably know that babies start to respond to smiles socially around two months, but the fascinating thing is even babies who are blind will smile around this time too. How are we genetically programmed to *smile?*

So questions like this will keep my motivation up all the way through my training and career. I have my own children who I think started my fascination with pregnancy, birth and the postnatal period, and this may help me relate to some clients, although we all experience these events differently.

I should also add that I'm good with my hands and quickly pick up skills, and I can't bear having an office job - I'm much better on my feet all day! So for all these reasons I think I would be an excellent candidate.

26. How would you act as an advocate for women?

This question addresses your ability to look at the challenges women might have getting the care they want, and how you would address these limitations. It hints at the midwifery role of normalising pregnancy and birth. Medical interventions like caesareans and assisted birth are becoming more common year on year. Some countries like America offer very medicalised care which appears to increase mortality and morbidity for mothers and newborns. This question is asking how much you know about these things, and whether you'd be able to make a difference to women in practice - quite an advanced question if you read into it!

This is a difficult question for me to answer as I am new to midwifery, but I do understand there are challenges for women to get the type of care they want. For instance, some hospitals don't have pools and many women want to labour or give birth in water. In these kind of situations I would try and ask managers if we could do something practical to allow pool birth - for instance, use blow up pools with the right health and safety measures in place. I think this is an example of being an advocate for women.

On a case by case basis, there might be women who have decided on care that from a medical point of view is not safe, or they might be encouraged to do something they are not comfortable with. This is a really difficult area to navigate, but I would always support women in their choices after I was sure they had all the information. I'd imagine these situations need experienced midwives' input, so although I would always fight for women's choices, I would try to learn as much as possible from mentors and midwives who I thought were doing an excellent job.

27. What do you plan to do within the next 5 years?

This question addresses how committed you are to your career choice. It is asking whether you see yourself heading towards a specialist role. Common pitfalls include: saying you have no idea what kind of midwife you'd make; saying you're not sure; or saying you will have to try midwifery out before knowing you're in it for the long haul.

Interviewers might be happier hearing you identify a few potential career paths you have interest in, or merely saying you are excited at the prospect of being that experienced. Note: you don't have to follow a career path just because you mentioned it once in an interview! Showing you have an interest in furthering your education and role after your training will be very attractive to interviewers. Talking about your specialist interest subject while answering this question would be excellent (you can find more information about specialist interest subjects on page 98).

I would perhaps be working towards a specialist role in midwifery.

I'm really interested in how to provide good care for women who are obese. I think it's a problem that will continue to be an issue in terms of resources and outcomes. I have a keen interest in why so many people find it hard to be in good shape, and I think midwives are well placed to improve matters. It would be really exciting to be a part of this.

28. Are your family supportive of your plans to become a midwife?

This question screens for candidates who do not have good support. This is a difficult question to answer without knowing your situation, but I will assume that if you are at this stage, you feel you have enough support to train as a midwife. Common mistakes would include seeming uncertain, or making light of your lack of support. It would be best to concentrate on the positives; remember most people's families will have some concerns about the course because it is very demanding. I have included two answers to cover both a candidate with excellent support, and a candidate with a more complicated story.

A] My family are very pleased I've found something I get so fired up over. They are proud I want to do something worthwhile. We have a realistic idea of this career choice - I know I will need their support, and they can see it's an investment in my future.

B] My partner was a bit sceptical at first; I think he
can't understand why anyone would want to work
around blood and body fluids! However he's getting
more interested when I'm reading midwifery
textbooks and forums. He has a busy job and I've
always had a busy job, so we've talked about how
we'd schedule special time together while I'm working
shifts. But we're quite used to working around each
other's schedules; I know it wouldn't work for some
couples, but it does for us. He likes seeing me so
excited over a prospective career choice.

29. How would you react to criticism from a qualified midwife which was heard by other students or professionals? How about in front of a client?

*This question addresses one of the key attributes an exceptional
candidate will have: resilience to criticism (more can be found in
the Chapter Five: "Above and Beyond"). As a student midwife
you must be able to take constructive criticism while being
resilient to unconstructive criticism. Poor responses would
include showing a tendency towards conflict, or an inability to
stand up for yourself if the criticism was unfair or
unprofessional.*

As part of any learning process, you need to be given
criticism. It's natural to not enjoy criticism, but it's
essential to improve, and I do want to be an excellent
practitioner. I can also understand that in a busy ward
situation, midwives might need to offer corrections in
front of other staff or even clients. I would try to
'take it on the chin'! And hopefully improve.

I imagine just like in any work setting however, there will be the odd time when mentors are not correct in their criticism and may even be unprofessional. In these situations I would try and take the midwife to one side and state my concerns, if I thought this would improve our relationship or my learning. I hope this wouldn't happen too often, but I do have a realistic idea of what working on a busy ward could be like.

30. Was there a specific experience that made you want to be a midwife?

This question appears to be more of a conversation starter between you and the interviewers. They may be looking at your passion for the career, or making sure your motivation is based on a real idea of the job and is sustainable. A common error would be describing a friend or family member's birth that was 'perfect' - it's not catastrophic to do this but a stronger answer would also address how you would cope with more difficult circumstances.

I haven't ever attended a birth and I can't put my finger on where my fascination started. However I took my time over deciding on a career path. I have a friend who is a midwife and a few who are nurses, and it seemed they had similar personalities and skills to me. Midwifery appeals to me more than nursing as it deals with well people; it seems like such a positive profession in that respect. I also find pregnancy and birth fascinating.

31. How did your work experience prepare you for a role as a midwife?

*This question wants you to identify skills that a midwife must
have, and show how your work experience started to develop
these skills for you.*

I worked in an elderly ward at the weekend for 6
months. I really enjoyed it in some ways, but it made
me realise I wouldn't want to be a nurse! However I
now have a basic idea of how a ward works, how to
do bed baths, help with personal hygiene and bed
changes and makes. I also understand that a lot of
people in hospital don't want to be there and often
just want a good listener. I think having basic ward
experience will be useful in terms of benefiting the
team right away - I can clean and make up rooms, and
know how meal systems work. I also think listening
skills and the ability to pick up skills through
observation will be very useful. One of the nurses
kindly showed me how to take a pulse, temperature
and blood pressure, so that's a good start as well!

I would have loved the opportunity to volunteer or
work at a maternity ward, but my local hospital were
not taking anyone on.

Analysis And Sample Answers: On Your Personal Opinions And Factual Knowledge About Midwifery And Related Topics

1. What do you think midwives do on a day to day basis? What do different types of midwives do?

Midwives look after women throughout the antenatal,
intrapartum and postnatal periods. They are experts in
normal pregnancy and birth. They have to know
when to refer women for medical care and how to
give emergency care. They also look after the
wellbeing of healthy newborns. They offer emotional
support and empowerment for women and their
families.

Different types of midwives might include specialists
in diabetes, pre-eclampsia, bereavement, mental
health, vulnerable women who need social work
input, HIV specialists and lactation consultants.

**2. If you were looking after a woman who refused
an important part of medical care, how would
you approach the subject?**

I respect the right of every woman to make decisions
about her care. I would give her all the information in
a format that she understood - for instance, if she
didn't speak English I would use a translation service,
or if she was young and having problems
understanding a lot of medical terminology, I would
try and get her good support and explain things in
terms she understood. I would also make sure she had
the best opinions available, for instance if I felt she
needed to see a consultant doctor I would try and
arrange that.

I would ask for help from my manager if it was a
difficult situation that might end in harm. I might talk
to a more experienced midwife who could advise me.
I know documenting things would be really important

in this kind of situation. I think it's really important to keep women 'on side' though, because I have heard of cases where women completely disengage from care, and this would obviously be the most unsafe scenario.

3. What barriers do you think midwives face in inner city areas? What about in rural areas?

Inner city areas probably have more socio-economic problems, for instance drug or alcohol abuse, non-English speaking women, refugees, women and families with limited money to spend on a good diet, and more people smoking. These would be barriers to care as they require more input on the part of midwives to get good outcomes.

Rural areas would probably have all these problems too, but less frequently. Other barriers might include clients feeling more isolated if they live very rurally, problems with driving a long way to women for intrapartum or postnatal care, or problems for women getting to hospital in labour.

4. What kind of other professionals do midwives work with?

They liaise with lots of professionals, including obstetricians, neonatal nurses, dieticians, social workers, sonographers, occupational therapists and more.

5. Midwives are very important in terms of women's health. What benefit do they have on society as a whole?

Midwives are present at the beginning of people's
lives, so can have an impact on the next generation.
For instance, improving women's diets, smoking
habits, drug and alcohol habits and way of life during
pregnancy can have a lasting effect on her child's life.
They also in my opinion have a very interesting job in
that they offer holistic care. They cover the medical
needs of women having normal pregnancies, but also
make sure their emotional and social needs are taken
care of. Having a confidence-building labour and
birth experience during which women feel able to
make their own decisions can be just the introduction
into motherhood that some women need. So
midwives can have a positive effect on society as a
whole by working in a grassroots manner, woman by
woman, pregnancy by pregnancy.

Midwives have been part of major health drives, for
instance in trying to reduce smoking and promote
breastfeeding. I know there is also a government drive
to allow midwives to 'deliver excellence' by 2020, and
midwives will in the future need to address the rising
intervention rate, rising number of women who have
complex medical needs, rising levels of obesity and so
on.

**6. How will you cope counselling or reassuring
frightened families or partners? What if their
concerns are irrational, for instance, they worry
that the baby isn't getting enough fluid
breastfeeding despite feeding going well?**

It's natural for families to be anxious about a loved one. However, their concerns will not always be helpful. I would try and put myself in their position - how would I feel if I had a similar concern about my sister or my daughter?

I would give them time to state their concerns, and I would listen to them to validate their importance. Then I might praise them for caring so much about the baby, and offer them evidence that all was well. I might also comment that lots of women give up breastfeeding through lack of confidence or feeling unsupported, and give them some written material or information on the massive benefits breastfeeding can have.

I think most people just want their concerns to be heard because they are worried some aspect of care has been overlooked.

7. Do you think having had children is an advantage as a midwife?

What an interesting question. Not necessarily. I'm sure some midwives benefit from the insight that having children gives them. Some midwives with children might have never laboured as they had caesareans births, which shows everyone's experience is different. I don't think you can assume personal experience of having children means you are better qualified as a midwife.

I think it's more important that midwives are caring and competent, and you can get to that position via all sorts of paths.

8. Why are midwives essential to women's health, as opposed to having nurses or doctors perform the same function?

Midwives appear to reduce the mortality and morbidity of mothers and their babies in lots of countries. I've read this is because they are specialists in normal birth and pregnancy, so reduce unnecessary interventions which can have bad side effects. I suspect this is also because they try to empower women to be in charge of their health and their babies' health.

Some argue that obstetricians and nurses have a different philosophy of care which is more medicalised. Midwives have experience with normal pregnancy and birth which means they are more able to keep women in a healthy, normal category unless absolutely necessary.

9. Women often have a birth partner with them during labour. What do you think their role is? How would you support them through all aspects of midwifery care?

Birth partners are very important to most women, and therefore are an important part of holistic midwifery care.

I know that birth partners can have an effect on outcomes; well supported women need less pain relief for example. Ideally women need to feel supported by their birth partner, though I understand this isn't always the case. I would try and involve birth partners through the pregnancy care, if this is what the client in question wants. Birth plans should be available to birth partners and they should have some idea of what might happen during labour and birth. I would try and give them the skills and confidence to help their loved one in labour. I expect it can sometimes be difficult to separate a woman's wants and needs from her birth partner's so this would need careful attention, and in a perfect world you would know the woman in question well so you could work this out. I think the main thing to remember here is something my mother taught me: 'calm is catching'. If you can get a woman's birth partner to be calm and confident, she is much more likely to be calm and able to cope with her labour.

10. What have you seen in the news recently in terms of midwifery? How do you think midwives are treated by the press?

Midwives being struck off the register is something that features in the media frequently. This is a hard thing to discuss with your interviewers, and if possible I would choose a different piece of media to comment on.

However, if an event like this has been publicised in the press before your interview, not mentioning the case may make it appear you are out of touch with current midwifery events. If this happens, I would comment that it's very difficult to know all the facts through the media, and ask for your interviewers'

*opinions. I would also comment that midwives seem to provoke
an inflammatory response in the press - new mothers and babies
coming to harm is something everyone gets emotional about and
therefore such stories get a lot of coverage, despite maternal and
neonatal mortality and morbidity decreasing in the UK every
year.*

*Commenting negatively on a midwife's practice might not be the
best thing to do as interviewers might feel you cannot judge when
you haven't trained yet. A safer yet still interesting topic might
be budget cuts in the NHS, a new piece of technology or study,
or an interesting human interest story. I have included two
answers, one to cover midwives being criticised in the press, one
on a different subject entirely.*

A] Well the press is full of that case of the midwife in
Cornwall who has been struck off the register. It
seems to be a topic that comes up a lot in the press,
despite the fact neonatal and maternal deaths keep
going down in the UK. I think it's a topic that sells a
lot of papers, as people find the death of a baby very
emotive. I feel very sorry for the families and
midwives involved, and I can't really comment on the
case because I don't have enough information and I
don't feel like it would be my place considering I
haven't even started training yet. I suppose it's just
inspiration to be extremely careful with the lives in
your care. The press seems to be very interested in
midwifery right now, and I'm sure there are lots of
theories as to why that is, but I think it's important to
acknowledge that the media exists to sell itself, so it's
not always real.

B] There was a very encouraging study commented about in a BBC news article. It summed up care in Scotland - I think 90% of women were really happy with their care. However it did find about a fifth of the women were left alone in labour at a time which made them feel worried. This might reflect staffing issues, and it also might reflect women's lack of confidence in birth as a process. It's hard to pick articles like this apart. I think it's important to recognise that the media exists to sell itself, and it will focus on statistics which appear worrying at times without there being a good reason to do so. I'd try to look at the studies themselves before coming to a conclusion.

I do think the current media attention to midwifery is very good in some ways; funding is likely to be channelled into maternity services if it is of public interest. It probably means I have lots of healthy competition in applying to be a midwife though!

11. What does normal/natural birth mean to you?

This question is really asking you what you know and what you think about the medicalisation of childbirth. In a nutshell, research and evidence suggests that normal, natural birth needs good teamwork from midwives, and women with a healthy attitude to birth and good support. Some experts claim that these things are far more important to normal birth and we should focus on them instead of medicalised aspects of care like IV drips and electronic fetal monitoring. Quite a juicy question! You don't have to have a clear opinion on this - it's a really

contentious issue. You just have to demonstrate you are aware
of the arguments and have thought about it.

I've had a good think about this as some of my
friends have had a birth needing forceps, but they still
describe their experience as a 'natural' birth. For the
women themselves I wonder if it matters if they say
'normal' or 'natural' when in fact they've had
intervention. Whatever makes them happy seems fine
to me; they're the ones who have to square
themselves with the experience.

I know there are some authors and activists who
would say normal birth hardly exists any more in
Western countries. I'm not sure what I think about
this; I think I need more information. But certainly I
think midwives have a big role to play in making sure
women have the best experience they can have.

I would say a caesarean is not a normal or natural
birth, but this doesn't mean it's a bad thing for all
women. Equally I would err on the side of saying
instrumental birth is not natural, but again, they've
saved a lot of lives so this doesn't necessarily mean
they are always bad.

I know the Royal College of Midwives has a
'campaign for normal birth' and it seems sensible to
get good natural practices into midwifery care as these
don't cost much, don't harm anyone, appear to
benefit mums and empower women to have the birth
they most want.

12. Do you think it's important midwifery has become a degree based programme?

This question is asking you whether you think it's important midwives are well educated, as opposed to just being able to do the physical side of the job. As you are talking to a university interviewer, it is probably best to say yes! A pitfall would be to say that midwives don't need much education, or saying midwifery just requires common sense.

I know that you could train as a midwife and just get a diploma up until recently. I'm sure there are lots of things I don't know about the changes to educating midwives.

It seems that a midwife really needs to be able to look at research and understand the political climate to be an advocate and truly work for women. An all-graduate workforce also helps the profession be credible I suppose, rightly or wrongly. I think education is a very good thing always, so I can't imagine many downsides to it being a degree based programme. Just as long as it doesn't become all academic - midwifery needs to be based in the real world, there's no point knowing lots of things about birth if you don't have the skills to act as a competent midwife!

13. Imagine you are a woman in labour. What are your needs? What is most important to you?

This question is judging your empathy, ability to anticipate needs, and your aptitude to an important part of being a midwife: intrapartum care.

I would want to feel I was being looked after by
someone who knew what they were doing. A skilled
person I felt safe around. I would want to be
respected and cared for. I would want my loved ones
nearby if I needed them. I would want to feel I had
choice in the kind of pain relief I had available, and
any interventions I needed. Most important to me
personally would be knowing the baby was doing well
and feeling that if something went wrong I would
have the right medical support. I would want dignity,
choice, and to feel listened to.

14. Breastfeeding can be a contentious issue. Can you describe some of the benefits and issues?

*This question is to assess your knowledge of the
breastfeeding/ bottle feeding choice women make, and the areas
of debate and emotion around the subject.*

The research suggests breastfeeding is the best
nutrition for a baby. It has important immunological
properties, decreases the risk of allergies, diabetes,
and obesity, and I've read that it can also positively
affect IQ.

However, many women don't want to breastfeed for
personal reasons- many feel uncomfortable because
breasts are linked to sex, or they think it's likely to
change their appearance, or they don't want to be
seen in public feeding. Because breastfeeding is so
important to some women because they feel closer to
their baby, or they maybe think every baby has a right
to be breastfed, the formula/breastfeeding question
can become a bit of an argument.

Breastfeeding can also be tricky to get right for some
women and might have painful aspects. It's also very
time consuming.

All in all I can imagine it's very rewarding helping
with breastfeeding, but also quite difficult sometimes
to support women with their choices with all the facts
and emotions involved.

**15. Homebirth can also be a contentious issue.
Can you describe some of the debate? What are
your personal ideas?**

*This is an interesting question. Many midwives have personal
beliefs that fall heavily for or against home birth. Common
pitfalls would include damning or praising homebirth without
going into any facts or opinions from the other side of the
argument.*

I know a few studies have found that homebirth for
normal, healthy women can be just as safe as hospital
birth. Women tend to labour better in a familiar
environment because that's how the hormones work.
They are more likely to listen to their bodies and do
their own thing, which can lead to better outcomes.

However, sometimes things go wrong during birth.
Obviously any midwife attending a homebirth would
be well trained in how to respond to an emergency
but emergencies do exist that are adversely affected
by being away from a hospital, for instance if a baby
needs complicated resuscitation.

I would say women need to be really well educated
about the risk factors and benefits and then make

their own minds up. It's then up to midwives to
support women to do what makes them comfortable
in labour. Just from personal experience, I think
sometimes if women come into hospital when they
don't want to, it can cause more problems, mental
and physical, than if they'd stayed at home. It's such a
personal choice.

16. How would you deal with difficult or aggressive clients or partners/families?

*This question is again checking you have thought through the
challenges that come with midwifery. Perhaps talk about a time
you've dealt with a situation like this, if you have applicable
experience.*

Pregnancy and birth are really emotional times for
loads of people. It can be scary, and life changing.
Therefore I can imagine some people kicking off - I
read something on a blog the other day that said
'birth brings out the best and the worst'. I would try
really hard to listen to their concerns and try to de-
escalate the situation. I've actually dealt with a
situation like this on the elderly ward I did work
experience on - one of the elderly women had a son
who was shouting at the staff because he thought his
Mum had been neglected.

The lady in question was actually just elderly and
confused - I won't go into the particulars but it wasn't
actually the staff's fault. I talked to him calmly and
quietly, then listened to all his concerns, and told him
if he wanted to complain to the manager I could help
with that process.

I also praised him for caring about his mother so
much, but told him we were very happy to listen to all
feedback and would change anything possible, and he
didn't need to raise his voice to be listened to. Luckily
he calmed down at this point and we were able to
reassure him that the care was good. I assume if he
had got violent or had continued to shout, we would
have called security.

I think the thing to remember here is although you
get one or two idiots around, mostly people are just
scared or feel they're not listened to if they're kicking
off - apologise and listen to them and they usually
come round.

17. What do you think about the rising caesarean rate?

*This question is similar to question 11 which dealt with normal
birth. You don't have to know all the facts and figures about
caesareans, just the basic debate about the medicalisation of
childbirth.*

I know the caesarean rate has been rising for a long
time, and medicalisation of childbirth is escalating in
most western countries. I think this is concerning
because it's so expensive and caesareans are massive
abdominal operations - it's not good to do these
things unless you really have to, to avoid infection
and complications.

However the maternal mortality and morbidity rate is
going down. So I think this is a really interesting,
important debate in maternity care which I don't have

enough information on to answer properly. But I would suggest midwives have a key role to play in getting women to have non medicalised birth as this is often what they prefer and often safer, and more life affirming for the women in question. I am talking generally, there will always be women who benefit from medicalised care, and it's great it's there and relatively safe when we need to use it.

18. Describe why prioritising privacy and dignity for clients is important

This question addresses your empathy towards the women who will be in your care.

Women should be comfortable telling their midwife intimate things about their health and lifestyle. Therefore midwives should be careful with women's privacy and dignity as they can feel their trust has been abused, say if you reveal information to a woman's family that she told you in confidence.

In labour women often want to remove clothes and get into different positions, and they might not think about this at the time, but looking back on the experience, they might well appreciate that the room wasn't full of people they didn't know or that someone covered them with a discrete towel or sheet. Dignity would also include not telling professionals who didn't need to know that the woman in question has had a sexually transmitted infection, or has a history of drug and alcohol use.

So essentially to make the woman's experience as
good as possible, and her care as effective as possible.

19. If you had to prioritise two main attributes a midwife should have, what would they be?

*This question assesses your ability to think on your feet and
asks for a basic understanding of the role of a midwife. There is
no need to overcomplicate this question; choose two excellent
attributes that midwives should have, for instance empathy,
professionalism, a careful nature, a feeling of privilege to work
with women going through pregnancy and birth, being calm,
organised, and passionate and so on.*

I think midwives first of all need to have the ability to
keep calm. Most women and families will get worried
or distressed about something during pregnancy, birth
or the postnatal period, and even if something's going
wrong, a calm attitude is going to have a positive
impact. Panicking might make things even more
dangerous, or a client even more worried.

I think midwives should always retain their passion
for the job. Midwifery is very demanding career and
many rely on them to give them good care; a passion
for looking after people during their path to
parenthood must be based on rock solid motivation
to do a good job for every woman.

20. Can you list some things you think would not take place in a normal labour?

*This question again asks about your knowledge of the
medicalisation of childbirth. This question is more difficult
however as it specifically asks you to state your opinion of what*

doesn't count as normal. Common mistakes candidates might make would be seeming judgemental of certain practices, or having no opinion at all, or not identifying key areas in which midwifery is over medicalised. I would state your opinion with a justification, but add that you have a lot more to learn on the subject.

I think some things should be understood to be medical interventions not needed in normal labour. I know the Royal College of Midwives suggest that CTGs are not good to use in normal low risk labour. It seems we pick up lots of problems that are not really problems if you know what I mean. I also know in some countries women as a matter of course have epidurals and IV fluids, which seems unnecessary in normal birth.

I know there's lots of evidence around which suggests normal, low risk labour and birth can't really be improved by medicine.

21. What is the biggest change in midwifery within the last forty years?

This question is asking what knowledge you have around midwifery in terms of history and politics. It's asking for an interesting insight. Good answers might include more available epidurals, more caesareans, more use of CTGs or Dads being present in the birth room.

I know episiotomies used to be routine for every woman, whether or not they needed them. I also know that steroids started to be used around 50 years ago to improve premature babies' lung function.

I think looking at everything I've read the biggest
change has been in women's expectations. It seems 40
years ago women were far more likely to follow a
parental model of care, and follow their doctor's
instructions. Today there is a lot of media focussed
around pregnancy and birth, along with lots of
activism. Women are far more likely to have a specific
birth plan with things they've chosen, like waterbirth,
standing birth, etc.

22. Should we have more male midwives?

*This is a fascinating question. 99.8 % of midwives are female
and there is no real conversation going on about the suitability
of men to be midwives. It is a question asking how much
reading around the subject you have done, and how deep your
thinking goes. It is also a question which addresses whether you
can talk about difficult topics within midwifery. I would talk
about inherent sexism, patient choice, possible religious reasons
a client would not want a male midwife, and how male
midwives might support birth partners well. It would also be
fine to present your own opinion here - it is not a topic which
many midwives have a good answer for. A common pitfall
would be coming across inherently sexist towards men
(remember many of your colleagues i.e. obstetricians,
anaesthetists, will be men who will look after your clients in
intimate ways). You should also try not to feel embarrassed by
the question as this looks like you are unable to talk about
complex issues!*

This is a really interesting question. I think male
midwives must be very brave, as midwifery is a female
dominated profession. It's such an unusual situation

as so many professions are all male, with women trying to break in: in this case it's reversed.

I think women and men are designed to work together. We often have different attributes, and together we can offer the complete package. So for this reason it might be really positive to support more male midwives to train.

However, some clients might feel uncomfortable with a male midwife, just like they might feel uncomfortable about having a male doctor. They might have suffered from sexual abuse from a man, may have religious beliefs which stop them being seen intimately by a male midwife, or just be unused to a male midwife. In these cases just like anything else, client choice should be respected. I imagine there would be plenty of women who wouldn't care what sex their midwife was, or might even prefer a male midwife.

I also think male midwives might be useful in supporting male birth partners and husbands. I know from personal experience partners can feel quite dominated by a female environment, so a male midwife might even things up a bit!

Analysis And Sample Answers: Scenario Based Questions

1. Tell me about different positions women may find useful in labour? What about for giving birth?

*This question is investigating how much reading you have done
and what you believe about low risk care. The medicalisation of
childbirth has meant women have started giving birth lying
down, which is a really difficult position working against gravity
and decreasing the diameter of the pelvic outlet. You can read
more about this medicalistion of childbirth process in terms of
positions at the excellent evidencebasedbirth.com:*
*www.evidencebasedbirth.com/what-is-the-evidence-for-pushing-
positions/*

I think it's important to listen to what a woman's
body is telling her to do. This is usually getting into
lots of upright positions, moving around and jiggling
the baby down into her pelvis. There are lots of tools
they can use like the birth pool which makes it easier
for them to get into different positions, birth balls,
leaning against their partner etc.

In terms of pushing I know it's traditional for women
to give birth lying down and this also means the
caregiver can see what's going on easily. However this
doesn't make good use of gravity and it's quite hard
to push that way. Upright positions or hands and
knees positions might be easier and more
comfortable.

**2. Jehovah's witness clients have a religious belief
that means they will not or cannot accept blood
products. How would you react looking after a
woman in your care who was dying through this
choice?**

*This question is looking at your ability to cope with and talk
about the darker side of midwifery.*

This would be a very, very hard situation. I would
need lots of support from colleagues I think.

Jehovah's witnesses I think usually have legal
paperwork that confirms they don't want a blood
transfusion and it would be really important to make
sure it was really what she wanted. You would have to
make sure she knew that this was the choice; a blood
transfusion or possibly dying.

I would try to look after all her other needs and make
sure it was the best care I could possibly offer without
a blood transfusion. However I would have to
honour her needs, although I'm sure I would find it
very emotional. I would then try and support the
family and the baby's needs as much as possible. I
would get their spiritual leaders involved if this was
what they wanted, and hope they made the best
decision for them.

**3. You are looking after a woman with social
services input. She has had her first two babies
taken into care because of drug use and a violent
home. She comes to see you pregnant with her
third child. How would you cope with the
situation?**

*This question is again asking you to consider the darker side of
midwifery and how you would cope personally. You don't have
to know exact procedure. Just state you would get help and
advice, and try to give the woman in question as much support
as possible to help her get the best outcome for her and her baby,
whether that means the baby being taken into care or her
parenting long term.*

I think there is a team I would need to liaise with - social workers and specialist midwives should be involved. However I would try to make the woman see I was on her side and I respected her - one of my core beliefs is that I am very lucky in my life and life choices, and it's not up to me to judge anyone else, as I could easily be in their position.

I would try to make her understand that I had to look after the safety of her baby, but that she had lots of resources at her disposal to try and help her keep the baby. I would also try and make it easy for her to get to appointments and work around her needs. I would also want to look into if she was currently being abused or if there were domestic violence issues as that would obviously have an impact on where the baby went when born.

4. How would you cope if a family member of yours commented adversely about a pregnant teenager in public?

This is a controversial question trying to work out if your professionalism would apply to your home life as well - this is of course a very important part of being a midwife and you should show you would uphold the reputation of the profession.

I would be furious. My reaction would depend on the circumstance.

If I hadn't started training as a midwife yet, I would be really angry and ashamed of any of my family behaving like this. In fact I think it's very unlikely they would behave in this manner. I would say something

like 'shame on you for being so judgemental, you
don't know anyone's situation from seeing them in
the street, so what gives you the right to be so
unpleasant?'

If it had been heard by the lady in question and I
thought it was appropriate, I would make my family
member apologise to her and I would wish her well.

If I was a training midwife or qualified, I would loudly
tell them everyone has their own life path to lead, and
it's not up to us to judge - and in fact my job is to
help people if they are in a difficult circumstance. In
private I would also remind them that I am likely to
care for pregnant women from our area and it's really
inappropriate to comment like that.

5. How would you make women feel comfortable to breastfeed in public, if you had unlimited resources?

*This is really a question about how midwives might have an
impact on public health campaigns, what you know about the
subject of breastfeeding, and if you have an ability to think
outside the box.*

It would be really good to do a public campaign on
breastfeeding with adverts on TV. There's a great
poem on breastfeeding by Hollie McNish who is a
poet and a mum - it went viral on YouTube. It would
make a fantastic TV campaign with very little extra
money needed. I would also try and provide special
rooms around town, in supermarkets and elsewhere
so women could have privacy if they wanted it. But

really I would try and make it normal culture for women to breastfeed in public.

Chapter Eight: Male Midwives In The Making

The Challenges You Might Face

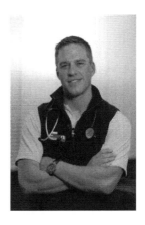

Well done for applying and wanting to be a midwife! You must be a guy who can think for himself because it's not a path that was laid out for you by society. I truly believe midwifery could benefit from some more male input, so welcome to the profession! This chapter will give you some bloke specific advice to help you become a successful applicant.

As a male midwife, your practice will be talked about by staff and patients alike. Male midwives become a bit notorious! You are likely to develop a respectful, hands off style of practice which many women appreciate and a lot of research appears to encourage. You are also likely to get lots of positive feedback as you'll be easy to spot and remember - though this works in reverse too when you have your bad days!

There is a chapter in *'Becoming a Midwife'* (Mander and Fleming, 2014) written by Dennis Walsh, a male midwife and researcher practicing in the UK. He has an interesting slant on being a male midwife, as he believes you have to thoroughly understand feminism and how midwifery relates to it to be a male midwife who practices with integrity. Whether you believe this is true or not is up to you but it's a good example of the slightly murky waters you will have to navigate to be a successful applicant.

It's good to remember that up until quite recently, it would have been culturally unacceptable for a man to be a nurse, or a gay couple to get married or adopt and these things are now protected in legislature. As a society we are moving forward and you are doing important work at the forefront.

You are in a similar position to anyone who has an ethnicity, sexual preference, sex or background that is perceived by many as at odds with the job you are applying for. You will therefore face many of the same challenges women have faced breaking into male dominated professions, or many ethnic groups have faced when applying for jobs.

Interviewers and others might have the following questions for you. You should think about your responses. My sample responses are at the end of this chapter. You can of course also use the sample panel interview questions/answers and other information, it's not gender specific! (I use the pronoun 'she' throughout the book just because 99% of midwives are female, but I don't mean to exclude you!)

What is your motivation to be a midwife?

How will you empathise with women as you are male?

How will you be able to make women feel at their ease, supported and cared for in labour?

How will you be able to remain confident in your practice if women question why you are a midwife who is male?

How will you deal with being 'notorious'?

How would you cope with a woman or her partner refusing your care because you are male?

I would just think hard about any concerns interviewers might have and be ready to head them off at the pass!

You also have an advantage in some ways because you can always remind your interviewer that you have thought out your career choice thoroughly - after all, applying to become a midwife as a man is not a run of the mill decision! Most interviewers will be very interested in what you have to say as a prospective male midwife.

• What is your motivation to be a midwife?

(The answer to the question wouldn't be any different if I were male - I repeat it here to aid your revision).

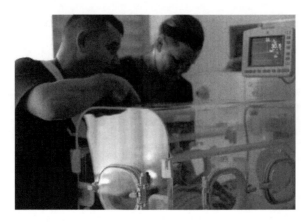

That's a huge question. I want to be a midwife because pregnancy, birth and the postnatal period fascinate me. I think midwives are onto something in the way they offer holistic care for women from social and emotional help all the way to the analysis of fetal hearts. I think what they offer amounts to true health care and helping women have their babies in an empowering way I think can affect whole societies. I am passionate, tough and very organised and I think my personality is suited towards ongoing challenges. I'm happiest when challenged.

How will you empathise with women as you are male?

I think empathy is based on understanding and motivation to offer support. I don't think this has that much to do with me being male - it might be slightly easier for someone with the same hormones and anatomy to empathise with a client in some situations, but not always - sometimes it might even lead to assumptions on the part of the midwife that they understand the client well without taking the time to really listen to them.

There are many childless female midwives who empathise with childbearing women really well. We all have our challenges in empathy and motivation, being male is not so different to other challenges.

I have also grown up with lots of women in my family I am very close to, and haven't felt it hard to empathise with them. I think some people have been culturally conditioned to think men can't empathise well with woman and I believe this simply isn't true.

How will you be able to make women feel at their ease, supported and cared for in labour?

In the same way as a female midwife would - by being competent, confident, and treating them with dignity. Examples would include making sure they are covered in labour to promote dignity, making sure they know they have a choice, offering true informed consent, and fulfilling the 'professional friendship' role of a midwife I have read about.

How will you be able to remain confident in your practice if women question why you are a midwife who is male?

I'm sure all healthcare professionals will be questioned by clients at some point. I imagine many women wouldn't have a problem at all being looked after by a male midwife. Others might have particular concerns, and I could address these by reassuring them I wanted to be a midwife because I am

fascinated with labour and birth, and think holistic
midwifery care is a brilliant model of care.

I would also remind them that there are plenty of
male obstetricians and gynaecologists - why do they
have concerns about me and not them?

Mostly however, I would try and make sure I was
personable and reassuring, which I'm sure would
allow most women to just get on with being cared for!

How will you deal with being 'notorious'?

I would try and ignore it as much as possible and get
on with my training. I imagine sometimes it would
help, other times it wouldn't, and overall it would
balance out.

**How would you cope with a woman or her
partner refusing your care because you are male?**

I imagine most midwives will have a conflict of
personalities at some point which will mean a client
asks not to be looked after by them. I would try and
work out from talking to other members of staff if it
was truly because I was male - and improve any
aspect of care they weren't happy with if applicable. If
it really was because I was male, I would go and look
after someone else!

There's nothing I can do to change being male, and I
understand some women will have a cultural or
religious reason for not wanting care from a male
midwife, or just not feel comfortable with a male
midwife. I would want women to make that decision

for themselves; I wouldn't want to look after a
woman who was really opposed to a male midwife
any more than they would want me looking after
them!

Good luck!

I'll finish with a quote from male midwife Dennis
Walsh:

*'I have no regret about my decision to become a midwife. It has
provided some of the most memorable experiences of my life, and
through it, I have met many remarkable people, both fellow
midwives and mothers. Of course, I have concerns about the
medicalisation of childbirth, the semi-autonomous, and not often
enough fully autonomous, nature of our role and the effects of an
institutional model on women. However, the privilege of
witnessing and attending physiological birth, with all its
challenge, courage and emotion, sustains me.'*

--Becoming a Midwife (Mander, 2009)

Chapter Nine: If You Didn't Get Offered A Place This Year

If You Didn't Get Offered a Place This Year: What it Says About You and Your Chances of Success

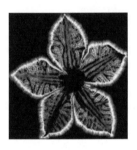

First of all, I'm sorry. It's always a bit painful when you've put a lot of effort into something and it hasn't worked out as planned. However, I'm sure you're wondering what this means in terms of you becoming a student midwife. Most people will be thinking - does this mean I'm not good enough? Did they see something that means I'm fundamentally not right to be a midwife?

Do you know what failing to get a place as a student midwife says about you? What it truly means? On almost all occasions?

ABSOLUTELY NOTHING!

The vast majority of the time you will simply have been up against too great a number of applicants, or your interviewers will have chosen 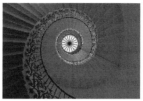 someone else based on a little more experience, or were perhaps looking for someone with a different personality or background to add diversity to their year group. These are all things you can't change.

It is HIGHLY UNLIKELY that your interviewers analysed your personality within 15 minutes of one-to-one interviewing, a personal statement and a few other tests and found you completely unsuitable. Don't take it personally; it's almost certainly not about you!

It hurts and it can knock your confidence. But you now have another year to put together a rock-solid application, and you have so much more experience to work with. This is a journey and it's a shame that you're going to have to take another shot at it - but there are two questions you need to ask yourself:

1. Will this affect me in 10 years' time?

It is highly unlikely that taking one or more years to commence your training will even be on your mind much in ten years' time. I can't imagine it occurring to you that often.

2. Is there anything you can do about it now?

No, you can't. The decision has been made and is out of your hands. Instead, concentrate on the things you can change:

Your 5 step plan to reapply:

1. Get feedback from the universities. Make notes, try to be stanch in your examination of their comments. If you don't understand what went wrong from their email or letter, get on the phone and have them explain. Be really truthful with yourself about what you could improve next time.

2. Get more experience. Try to talk to more midwives. Have a look at the experience section on page 15 for ideas.

3. Get onto 'The Secret Community for Midwives on the Making' on Facebook, and have a chat with others who didn't get in. Get some support, you deserve it, it's a competitive midwifery world out there.

4. Have another look at Chapter Five: *"Above and Beyond"*.

5. Use all your experience to reapply next year!

Now I know some of you will be shaking your heads and thinking 'no, actually, I'm rubbish, I'll never do it'…but the thing is, by reading this book, you are showing your enthusiasm and increasing your knowledge of midwifery to the point where I don't think you fall into this category.

If you have read this far, I think it's highly unlikely that you're unsuited to midwifery.

If you have researched how to interview, you fall into a small group of candidates that are very committed and clued up.

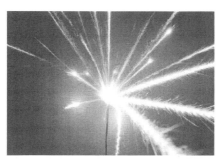

Just to reassure you - some of the best midwives I have ever worked with didn't get in first time. They are not embarrassed about it, and some even feel the extra year or so meant they were able to get more out of their training and offer better care to women.

Do you have a dream? Don't let someone, even a trained and experienced midwife decide you are not going to get onto a course. It's your life and your ambitions at stake - and besides, are you really going to let the profession miss out on such an excellent, committed prospective midwife?

I am going to finish with one of the most inspirational quotes I know of:

'Far better is it to dare mighty things, to win glorious triumphs, even though checkered by failure... than to rank with those poor spirits who neither enjoy nor suffer much, because they live in a gray twilight that knows not victory nor defeat.'

Theodore Roosevelt

CHAPTER NINE: IF YOU DIDN'T GET OFFERED A PLACE THIS YEAR

Good luck!

Congratulations!

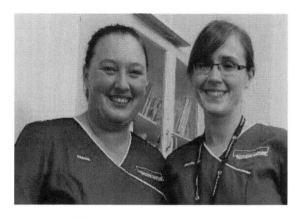

If you've followed the advice in this book, you should have a personal statement that will show insight and intelligence, an ability to interview well even under pressure, and an impressive knowledge of midwifery. You will have processed a lot of information over a short amount of time and learnt to apply it. You will have improved your chances of getting into your dream profession and working as a midwife no end. But more than this, **you will be a more able student midwife as soon as your feet hit the deck.**

I worked with a client this year from the beginning to the end of her application process (something I love to do). Her personal statement increased in quality to the point where she sounded like a midwife already. She started to understand what it really means to be a midwife, and did fantastically in her interview.

This is the real secret of preparing: learn to think like a midwife, and you will interview well, not through tricks or deceiving your interviewers, but by being able to get on the same wavelength as them. With this knowledge under your belt, you will be a student midwife I'd be proud to work with from the moment you enrol.

This is life changing stuff you're launching yourself into. It's not like you've seen on *'One Born Every Minute'* or *'Call The Midwife'*. It's a lot tougher - and a lot better.

Midwifery is frustrating, demanding, and sometimes even scary. But it's also life-changing, life-affirming and life-expanding. I hope I've got you to understand this. If you have, and you're up to the challenge, as a profession we're lucky to have you applying to be a midwife! I look forward to you joining us.

--Ellie Durant, from MidwifeDiaries.com

Index

A

Above And Beyond, 96
Access to Higher Education, 14, 58, 63

B

breastfeeding, 16, 29, 38, 40, 55, 87, 147, 200-201, 208-209, 220
burning out, 55

C

CEMACE, 102
check midwifery is right for you, 4
Cochrane, 59, 64-65, 89, 101-102, 141, 170
Computer, 18, 100
constructive criticism, 97, 104, 105, 195

D

day before your interview, 95
Department of Health, 86
DOPE, 73-74, 80, 114, 142
dyscalculia, 116
dyslexia, 34, 116

E

emotionally demanding, 143, 174

Entry grades, 13
Equality Philosophy, 79
Essay exams, 119
Essays, 135, 159
Eye contact, 84

G

Google Books, 19
Google Scholar, 19, 100
Group interviews, 110

H

hobbies, 43, 56

I

If You Didn't Get Offered a Place, 229
Ina May Gaskin, 46, 54, 170
Introverts, 73
IT skills, 145, 185-186

J

Jehovah's witness, 148, 217
journals, 19, 29, 37, 46, 52, 84, 120-121, 170, 191

L

Language comprehension, 122
legal, 17, 39, 85-86, 143, 175, 176, 218

Literacy Tests, 119, 135, 159

M

Male midwives, 222
Mature Student, 58
Michel Odent, 59, 65

N

neuro-linguistic programming,
    75, 76
NICE, 84, 86, 89, 101, 141
Numeracy Tests, 117, 124, 149
Nursing and Midwifery
    Council, 9, 39, 85, 89, 117

O

organisational skills, 35, 63

P

Panel Interview, 71, 81, 141,
    169
portfolio, 99, 106, 107
Posture, 83
Power Posing, 77, 80
Presentations, 114
prioritise, 43, 148, 213

Q

quote, 30, 41, 58, 61-62, 73,
    100, 122, 228
Quotes, 41

R

recently left full time
    education, 56
References, 13

Resilience, 104
Royal College of Midwives, 19,
    20, 28, 32, 86, 101, 206,
    214
Royal College of Obstetricians
    and Gynaecologists, 19,
    101

S

self-belief, 63
social media, 16
Specialist Interest Subject, 98
structure, 25, 38, 162, 172
Swearing, 93, 120

T

textbooks, 121
The National Institute for
    Health and Care
    Excellence, 86
The Secret Community For
    Midwives in the Making,
    95, 103, 231
transferable skills, 24, 34, 66,
    107, 110, 142, 171

U

UCAS Extra, 22, 110
UCAS, 12, 22,-23, 26, 36, 43
unsocial hours, 11, 143, 144,
    170, 176, 183

V

Visualisation, 76

W

Wikipedia, 19, 20, 85

work/life balance, 11, 43, 47,
    55-57, 88

Printed in Great Britain
by Amazon.co.uk, Ltd.,
Marston Gate.